SAFE MEDS
AN INTERACTIVE GUIDE TO
SAFE MEDICATION PRACTICE

prepared by

Peggy Przybycien, RN, MSN
Associate Professor of Nursing
Onondaga Community College
Syracuse, New York

software design and development by

Wolfsong Informatics, LLC
Tucson, Arizona

reviewed by

Kathleen Gutierrez, PhD, RN, ANP, CS
Denver, Colorado

Gina Long, RN, DNSc
Flagstaff, Arizona

Susan C. deWit, MSN, RN, CNS, PHN
Los Alamos, California

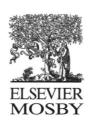

ELSEVIER
MOSBY

ELSEVIER
MOSBY

11830 Westline Industrial Dr.
St. Louis, Missouri 63146

Notice

Medication administration is an ever-changing field. Standard safety precautions must be followed, but as
new research and clinical experience broaden our knowledge, changes in treatment and drug therapy may
become necessary or appropriate. Readers are advised to check the most current product information provided by the manufacturer of each drug to be administered to verify the recommended dose, the method and
duration of administration, and contraindications. It is the responsibility of the licensed prescriber, relying
on experience and knowledge of the patient, to determine dosages and the best treatment for each individual
patient. Neither the publisher nor the author assumes any liability for any injury and/or damage to persons
or property arising from this publication.

International Standard Book Number 0-323-02766-0

Acquisitions Editor: *Tom Wilhelm*
Senior Developmental Editor: *Lauren Borstell*
Publishing Services Manager: *Gayle May*
Project Manager: *JoAnn Amore*
Cover Art: *Paula Ruckenbrod*

Printed in the United States of America

Last digit is the print number: 9   8   7   6   5   4   3   2   1

Contents

Getting Started

GETTING SET UP

■ **MINIMUM SYSTEM REQUIREMENTS**

PC

Windows XP, 2000, 98, ME, NT 4.0 (Recommend Windows XP/2000)
Pentium III processor (or equivalent) @ 600 MHz (Recommend 800 MHz or better)
128 MB of RAM (Recommend 256 MB or more)
800 x 600 screen size (Recommend 1024 x 768)
Thousands of colors
12x CD-ROM drive
Soundblaster 16 soundcard compatibility
Stereo speakers or headphones

Note: *Safe Meds* for Windows will require a minimal amount of disk space to install icons and required dll files for Windows 98/ME.

MACINTOSH®

MAC OS X (10.2 or higher)
Apple Power PC G3 @ 500 MHz or better
128 MB of RAM (Recommend 256 MB or more)
800 x 600 screen size (Recommend 1024 x 768)
Thousands of colors
12x CD-ROM drive
Stereo speakers or headphones

■ RUNNING SAFE MEDS

WINDOWS™

1. Install
   a. Insert the *Safe Meds* CD-ROM.
   b. Inserting the CD should automatically bring up the setup screen if the current product is not already installed.
      (1) If the setup screen does not appear automatically (and *Safe Meds* has not been installed already), navigate to the "My Computer" icon on your desktop or in your Start menu.
      (2) Double-click on your CD-ROM drive.
      (3) If installation does not start at this point:
         (a) Click the **Start** icon on the taskbar and select the **Run** option.
         (b) Type d:\setup.exe (where "d:\" is your CD-ROM drive) and press **OK**.
         (c) Follow the onscreen instructions for installation.
   c. Follow the onscreen instructions during the setup process.

2. Start
   a. Double-click on the ***Safe Meds*** icon located on your desktop.
   b. Or navigate to the program via the Windows Start menu.

   NOTE: Windows 98/ME will require you to restart your computer before running the *Safe Meds* program.

MACINTOSH®

1. Insert the *Safe Meds* CD in the CD-ROM drive. The disk icon will appear on your desktop.

2. Double-click on the disk icon.

3. Double-click on the SAFEMEDS_MAC run file.

   NOTE: *Safe Meds* for Macintosh does not have an installation setup and can only be run directly from the CD.

PRINTING

If you experience any problems with printing the evaluations, please verify that you have the latest drivers for your printer. Some machines may experience trouble printing. It is suggested that printing be done only from recommended systems.

TRADEMARKS

Windows™ is a registered trademark.

■ **SAFE MEDS**

Welcome to *Safe Meds*, Pacific View Regional Hospital. Pacific View Regional hospital is a multifloored institution comprising the following nursing units:

- Obstetrics Unit
- Pediatrics Unit
- Medical-Surgical Unit
- Skilled Nursing Unit

Within the simulation, you will care for realistic patients as a student nurse. As you care for your patients, you will have access to all of the patient's medical records, conduct physical assessments, and administer medication to patients. At the end of your shift, you will be provided with an evaluation of your work with the patients you cared for.

■ **TECHNICAL SUPPORT**

Technical support for this product is available at no charge by calling the Technical Support Hotline between 9 a.m. and 5 p.m. (Central Time), Monday through Friday. Within the United States, call 1-800-692-9010. Outside the United States, call 314-872-8370.

ACCESSING SAFE MEDS FROM EVOLVE

The product you have purchased is part of the Evolve family of online courses and learning resources. Please read the following information completely to get started.

1. **If your course is being led by an instructor:**

   A. **System**
   Find out what system your instructor is hosting the course on. Evolve courses can be run on a variety of systems, and your instructor will decide which one is right for your course.

   B. **User Name and Password**
   Your instructor will provide you with the user name and password needed to access the system where the course is located.

   C. **Login Instructions**
   If your instructor's course is being hosted on the *Evolve Learning System*, please see p. 9 for instructions on how to log in. If your course is located on a different system, your instructor will provide information on how to log in.

   D. **Access Code**
   You will need the access code located on the inside of the front cover of this workbook when you first access the course, regardless of what system the course is located on. When you are prompted, enter the code exactly as it appears.

2. **If you plan to take the course on your own** (Note: By taking the course independently, you will not have an instructor to help you. You will have 12 months from the date you are enrolled to complete the course):

   A. **System**
   All independent learners are enrolled in a course hosted on the *Evolve Learning System.*

   B. **Self-Enrollment**
   Please see p. 9 for instructions on how to self-enroll for the course.

   C. **User Name and Password**
   If you don't have an existing Evolve account, you will be able to create one during the self-enrollment process.

   D. **Login Instructions**
   See p. 9 for instructions on how to log in to the *Evolve Learning System.*

   E. **Access Code**
   You will need the access code located on the inside of the front cover of this workbook when you first access the course. When you are prompted, enter the code exactly as it appears.

TECHNICAL REQUIREMENTS

To use an Evolve course, you will need access to a computer that is connected to the Internet and equipped with web browser software that supports frames. For optimal performance, it is recommended that you have speakers and use a high-speed Internet connection. However, slower dial-up modems (56 K minimum) are acceptable.

Screen Settings

For best results, your computer monitor resolution should be set at a minimum of 800 x 600. The number of colors displayed should be set to "thousands or higher" (High Color or 16 bit) or "millions of colors" (True Color or 24 bit).

Windows™

1. From the **Start** menu, select **Control Panel** (on some systems, you will first go to **Settings**, then to **Control Panel**).
2. Double-click on the **Display** icon.
3. Click on the **Settings** tab.
4. Under **Screen area** use the slider bar to select **800 by 600 pixels**.
5. Access the **Colors** drop-down menu by clicking on the down arrow.
6. Select **High Color (16 bit)** or **True Color (24 bit)**.
7. Click on **OK**.
8. You may be asked to verify the setting changes. Click **Yes**.
9. You may be asked to restart your computer to accept the changes. Click **Yes**.

Macintosh®

1. Select the **Monitors** control panel.
2. Select **800 x 600** (or similar) from the **Resolution** area.
3. Select **Thousands** or **Millions** from the **Color Depth** area.

Web Browsers

Supported web browsers include Microsoft Internet Explorer (IE) version 5.0 or higher and Netscape version 4.5 or higher. *Note that Netscape version 6.0 is not supported at this time, although versions 6.2 and higher are supported.*

If you use America Online (AOL) for web access, you will need AOL version 4.0 or higher and IE 5.0 or higher. Do not use earlier versions of AOL with earlier versions of IE, because you will have difficulty accessing many features.

For best results with AOL:
- Connect to the Internet using AOL version 4.0 or higher.
- Open a private chat within AOL (this allows the AOL client to remain open, without asking whether you wish to disconnect while minimized).
- Minimize AOL.
- Launch a recommended browser.

Whichever browser you use, the browser preferences must be set to enable cookies and Java/JavaScript and the cache must be set to reload every time.

Enable Cookies

Browser	Steps
Internet Explorer 5.0 or higher	1. Select **Tools**. 2. Select **Internet Options**. 3. Select **Security** tab. 4. Make sure **Internet** (globe) is high-lighted. 5. Select **Custom Level** button. 6. Scroll down the **Security Settings** list. 7. Under **Cookies** heading, make sure **Enable** is selected. 8. Click **OK**.
Internet Explorer 6.0	1. Select **Tools**. 2. Select **Internet Options**. 3. Select **Privacy** tab. 4. Use the slider (slide down) to **Accept All Cookies**. 5. Click **OK**. -OR- 4. Click the **Advanced** button. 5. Click the check box next to **Override Automatic Cookie Handling**. 6. Click the **Accept** buttons under **First-party Cookies** and **Third-party Cookies**. 7. Click **OK**.
Netscape Communicator or Navigator 4.5 or higher	1. Select **Edit**. 2. Select **Preferences**. 3. Click **Advanced**. 4. Click **Accept all cookies**. 5. Click **OK**.
Netscape Communicator or Navigator 6.1 or higher	1. Select **Edit**. 2. Select **Preferences**. 3. Select **Privacy & Security**. 4. Select **Cookies**. 5. Select **Enable All Cookies**.

Enable Java

Browser	Steps
Internet Explorer 5.0 or higher	1. Select **Tools**. 2. Select **Internet Options**. 3. Select the **Advanced** tab. 4. Locate **Microsoft VM**. 5. Make sure the **Java console enabled** and **Java logging enabled** boxes are checked. 6. Click **OK**. 7. Restart your computer if you checked the **Java console enabled** box.
Netscape Communicator or Navigator 4.5 or higher	1. Select **Edit** 2. Select **Preferences**. 3. Select **Advanced**. 4. Make sure the **Enable Java** and **Enable JavaScript** boxes are checked. 5. Click **OK**.

Set Cache to Always Reload a Page

Browser	Steps
Internet Explorer 5.0 or higher	1. Select **Tools**. 2. Select **Internet Options**. 3. Select the **General** tab. 4. Select **Settings** from within the **Temporary Internet Files** section. 5. Select the **Every visit to the page** button. 6. Click **OK**.
Netscape Communicator or Navigator 4.5 or higher	1. Select **Edit** 2. Select **Preferences**. 2. Click the **+** or **→** icon next to the **Advanced** to see more options. 3. Select **Cache**. 4. Select the **Every time** button at the bottom. 5. Click **OK**.

Plug-Ins

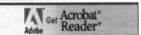 **Adobe Acrobat Reader**—With the free Acrobat Reader software you can view and print Adobe PDF files. Many Evolve products offer student and instructor manuals, checklists, and more in this format!

Download at: http://www.adobe.com

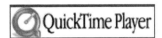 **Apple QuickTime**—Install this to hear word pronunciations, heart and lung sounds, and many other helpful audio clips within Evolve Online Courses!

Download at: http://www.apple.com

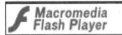 **Macromedia Flash Player**—This player will enhance your viewing of many Evolve web pages, as well as educational short-form to long-form animation within the Evolve Learning System!

Download at: http://www.macromedia.com

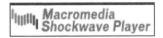 **Macromedia Shockwave Player**—Shockwave is best for viewing the many interactive learning activities within Evolve Online Courses!

Download at: http: //www.macromedia.com

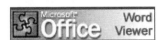 **Microsoft Word Viewer**—With this viewer Microsoft Word users can share documents with those who don't have Word, and users without Word can open and view Word documents. Many Evolve products have testbank, student and instructor manuals, and other documents available for downloading and viewing on your own computer!

Download at: http://www.microsoft.com

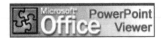 **Microsoft PowerPoint Viewer**—View PowerPoint 97, 2000, and 2002 presentations even if you don't have PowerPoint with this viewer. Many Evolve products have slides available for downloading and viewing on your own computer!

Download at: http://www.microsoft.com

SUPPORT INFORMATION

Live support is available to customers in the United States and Canada from 7:30 a.m. to 7:00 p.m. (Central Time), Monday through Friday by calling, **1-800-401-9962**. You can also send an email to evolve-support@elsevier.com.

There is also **24/7 support information** available on the Evolve website (http://evolve.elsevier.com), including:

- Guided Tours
- Tutorials
- Frequently Asked Questions (FAQs)
- Online Copies of Course User Guides
- And much more!

LOGIN INSTRUCTIONS

1. Go to the Evolve student page (http://evolve.elsevier.com/student).

2. Enter your user name and password in the **Login to My Evolve** area and click the **Login** button.

3. You will be taken to your personalized **My Evolve** page, where your course will be listed in the **My Courses** module.

SELF-ENROLLMENT INSTRUCTIONS

Important Note: These instructions apply only to individuals who are taking the course on their own. Remember that if you take the course independently, you will not have an instructor to help you. You will have 12 months from the date you are enrolled to complete the course.

1. Go to: http://evolve.elsevier.com/SafeMeds

2. Under the Online Course heading, click on the *Self-Study Student? Enroll Here* option. This will launch the Enrollment Wizard for your course.

3. Complete the Enrollment Wizard. During this process you will create an Evolve user name and password, you will be asked to provide identifying information about yourself, and will need to provide the access code from the inside front cover of this workbook.

4. Once the Wizard has been completed, you will be able to log in to your Evolve account and begin your online course immediately.

A QUICK TOUR

Welcome to *Safe Meds: An Interactive Guide to Safe Medication Practice*, a virtual hospital setting where you can learn to make decisions related to safe medication practice using simulated patients and commonly used health care records.

The virtual hospital, Pacific View Regional Hospital, has four nursing floors (Medical-Surgical, Obstetrics, Pediatrics, and Skilled Nursing) with realistic architecture and access to patient rooms, a Nurses' Station, and a Medication Room.

■ HOW TO SIGN IN

- Enter your name on the Student Nurse identification badge.
- Select a nursing floor—Medical-Surgical, Obstetrics, Pediatrics, or Skilled Nursing—by clicking the down arrow next to **Select Floor**. From the drop-down menu, highlight and click the floor you wish to work on. (For this quick tour, choose **Medical-Surgical**.)
- Now click the down arrow next to **Select Period of Care**. This drop-down menu gives you four periods of care from which to choose. In Periods of Care 1 through 3, you can actively engage in patient assessment, entry of data in the electronic patient record (EPR), and medication administration. Period of Care 4 presents the day in review. Highlight and click the appropriate period of care. (For this quick tour, choose **Period of Care 2**.)
- Click **Go** in the lower right side of the screen.
- This takes you to the Patient List screen (see example on next page). Only the patients on the floor you choose (Medical-Surgical) are available. Note that the virtual time is provided in the box at the lower left corner of the screen (1115, since we chose Period of Care 2).

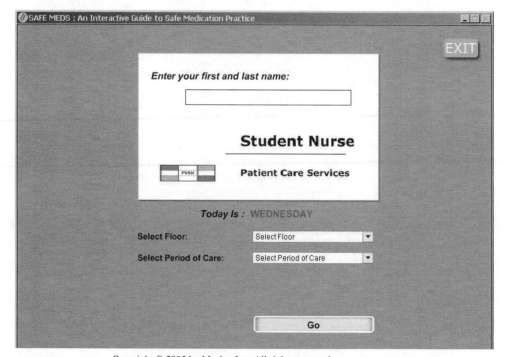

■ HOW TO SELECT A PATIENT

- You can choose one or more patients to work with from the Patient List by clicking the box to the left of the patient name(s). (In order to receive a scorecard for a patient, the patient must be selected before proceeding to the Nurses' Station.)
- Click on **Get Report** to the right of the medical records number (MRN) to view a summary of the patient's care during the 12-hour period before your arrival on the unit.
- Click on **Go to Nurses' Station** in the right lower corner.

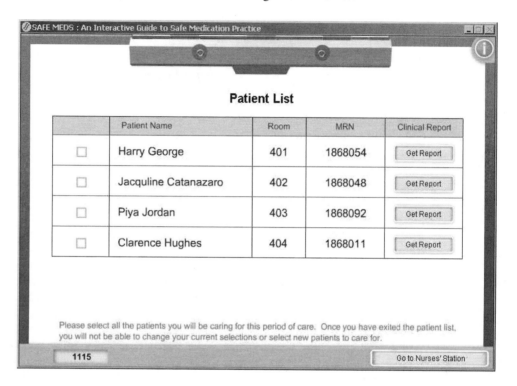

■ PATIENT LISTS

MEDICAL-SURGICAL UNIT

Harry George (Room 401)
Osteomyelitis—A middle-aged Caucasian male admitted from a homeless shelter with an infected leg. He has complications of type 2 diabetes mellitus, alcohol abuse, nicotine addiction, poor pain control, and complex psychosocial issues.

Jacquline Catanazaro (Room 402)
Asthma—A middle-aged Caucasian female admitted with an acute asthma exacerbation and suspected pneumonia. She has complications of chronic schizophrenia, noncompliance with medication therapy, obesity, and herniated disc.

Piya Jordan (Room 403)
Bowel obstruction—An older Asian female admitted with a colon mass and suspected adenocarcinoma. She undergoes a right hemicolectomy. This patient's complications include atrial fibrillation, hypokalemia, and symptoms of meperidine toxicity.

Clarence Hughes (Room 404)
Degenerative joint disease—An older African-American male admitted for a left total knee replacement. His preparations for discharge are complicated by the development of a pulmonary embolus and the need for ongoing intravenous therapy.

OBSTETRICS UNIT

Dorothy Grant (Room 201)
30-week intrauterine pregnancy—A young multiparous Caucasian female admitted with abdominal trauma following a domestic violence incident. Her complications include preterm labor.

Stacey Crider (Room 202)
27-week intrauterine pregnancy—A young Native American primigravida admitted for intravenous tocolysis, bacterial vaginosis, and poorly controlled insulin-dependent gestational diabetes.

SKILLED NURSING UNIT

William Jefferson (Room 501)
Alzheimer's disease—An elderly African-American male admitted for stabilization of type 2 diabetes mellitus and hypertension following a recent acute care admission for a urinary tract infection and sepsis. His complications include episodes of acute delirium.

Kathryn Doyle (Room 503)
Rehabilitation post-left hip replacement—An elderly Caucasian female admitted following a complicated recovery from an ORIF. Her complications include malnutrition, depression, unstable family dynamics (placing her at risk for elder abuse), and the onset of pneumonia.

Delores Gallegos (Room 502)
Congestive heart failure—An elderly Hispanic female admitted with progressive dyspnea at rest and the need for medication adjustment. This patient's complications include activity intolerance, poor dietary compliance, obesity, and dermatitis.

PEDIATRICS UNIT

George Gonzales (Room 301)
Diabetic ketoacidosis—An 11-year-old Hispanic male admitted for stabilization of blood sugars and diabetic reeducation associated with his diagnosis of type 1 diabetes mellitus. This patient's poor compliance with insulin therapy and dietary regime have resulted in frequent and repeated hospital admissions for DKA.

Tommy Douglas (Room 302)
Traumatic brain injury—A 6-year-old Caucasian male transferred from the Pediatric Intensive Care Unit in preparation for organ donation. This patient is status post-ventriculostomy with negative intracerebral blood flow and requires extensive hemo-dynamic monitoring and support along with compassionate family care.

■ HOW TO FIND A PATIENT'S RECORDS

NURSES' STATION

Within the Nurses' Station, you will see:

1. A clipboard that contains the patient list for that floor.
2. A chart rack with patient charts labeled by room number, a notebook labeled Kardex, and a notebook labeled MAR (Medication Administration Record).
3. A desktop computer with access to the Electronic Patient Record (EPR).
4. A tool bar across the top of the screen that can also be used to access the Patient List, EPR, Chart, MAR, and Kardex. This tool bar is also accessible from the patient room.
5. A Drug Guide containing information about the medications you are able to administer to your patients.

As you run your cursor over an item, it will be highlighted. To select an item, simply click on it. As you use these resources, you will always be able to return to the Nurses' Station by clicking on the **Return to Nurses' Station** bar located in the right lower corner of your screen.

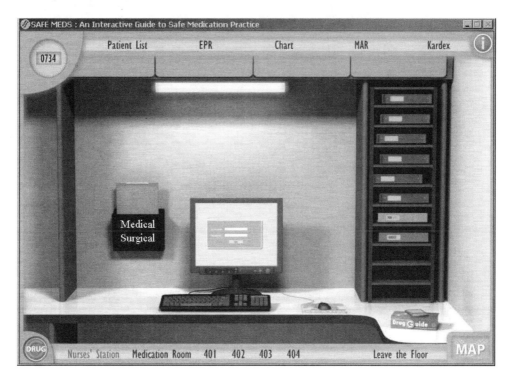

ELECTRONIC PATIENT RECORD (EPR)

The EPR can be accessed from the computer in the Nurses' Station and the also from the EPR icon located in the tool bar at the top of your screen. To access a patient's EPR:
- Click on either the computer screen or the **EPR** icon.
- Your user name and password are automatically filled in.
- Click on **Login** to enter the EPR.

The EPR used in Pacific View Regional Hospital represents a composite of commercial versions being used in hospitals. You can access the EPR:
- for a patient (by room number).
- to review existing data.
- to enter data you collect while working with a patient.

The EPR is updated daily, so no matter what day or part of a shift you are working, there will be a current EPR with the patient's data from the past days of the current hospital stay. This type of simulated EPR allows you to examine how data for different attributes have changed over time, as well as to examine data for all of a patient's attributes at a particular time. The EPR is fully functional (as it is in a real-life hospital). You can enter such data as blood pressure, breath sounds, and certain treatments. The EPR will not, however, allow you to enter data for a previous time period. Use the arrows at the bottom of the screen to move forward and backward in time.

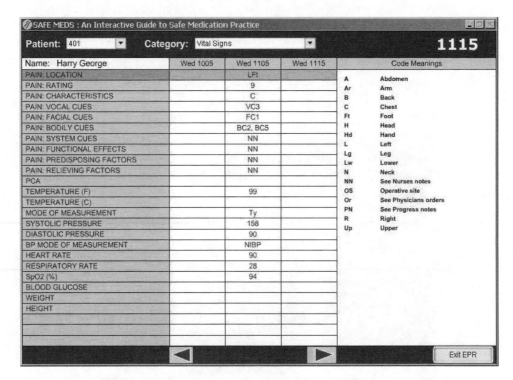

At the top of the EPR screen, you can choose patients by their room numbers. In addition, you have access to 17 different categories of patient data. To change patients or data categories, click the down arrow to the right of the room number or category.

The categories of patient data are:
- Vital Signs
- Respiratory
- Cardiovascular
- Neurologic
- Gastrointestinal
- Excretory
- Musculoskeletal
- Integumentary
- Reproductive
- Psychosocial
- Wounds and Drains
- Activity
- Hygiene and Comfort
- Safety
- Nutrition
- IV
- Intake and Output

Remember, each hospital selects its own codes. The codes in the Pacific View Regional Hospital may be different from ones you have seen in clinical rotations that have computerized patient records. Take some time to acquaint yourself with the codes. Within the Vital Signs category, click on any item in the left column (e.g., heart rate). In the far-right column, you will see a list of code meanings for the possible findings and/or descriptors for that assessment area.

You will use the codes to record the data you collect as you work with patients. Click on the box in the last time column to the right of the data and wait for the code meanings applicable to that entry. Select the code to describe your assessment findings and type it in the box. Once the data are typed in this box, they are entered into the patient's record for this period of care only.

To leave the EPR, click on **Exit EPR** in the bottom right corner of the screen.

CHARTS

To access patient charts, either click on the **Chart** icon at the top of your screen or anywhere within the chart rack to the right of the computer in the Nurses' Station. (Note: For chart access, be sure to click on the top part of the rack with the gray notebooks. The bottom two notebooks are for the MAR and Kardex.) When the close-up view appears, the charts are labeled by room number. To open a chart, click on the room number of the patient whose chart you wish to view. The patient's name and allergies will appear, along with a list of tabs on the right side of the screen, allowing you to view the following data:

- Allergies
- Physician's Orders
- Physician's Notes
- Nurse's Notes
- Laboratory Reports
- Diagnostic Reports
- Surgical Reports
- Consultations

- Patient Education
- History and Physical
- Nursing Admission
- Expired MARs
- Consents
- Mental Health
- Admissions
- Emergency Department

Information appears in real time. The entries are in reverse chronological order, so use the down arrow at the right side of the chart page to scroll down to view previous entries. Flip from tab to tab to view multiple data fields or click on the **Return to Nurses' Station** bar in the lower right corner of the screen to exit the chart.

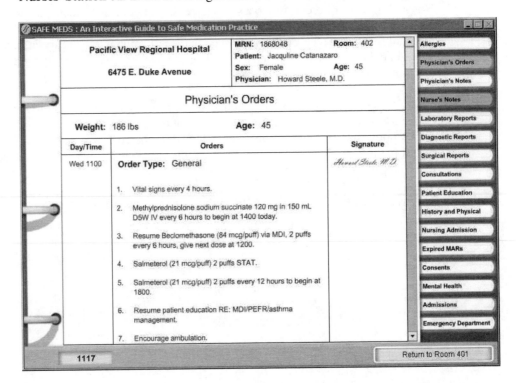

MEDICATION ADMINISTRATION RECORD (MAR)

The MAR icon located in the tool bar at the top of your screen accesses current 24-hour medications for each patient. Click on the icon and the MAR opens. (Note: You can also access the MAR by clicking on the blue MAR notebook in the book rack to the right of the computer.) Tabs on the right side of the screen allow you to select patients by room number. Be careful to make sure you select the correct tab number for *your* patient rather than simply reading the first record that appears after the MAR opens. Each MAR sheet lists the following:

- Medications
- Route and dosage of medications
- Times of administration of medication

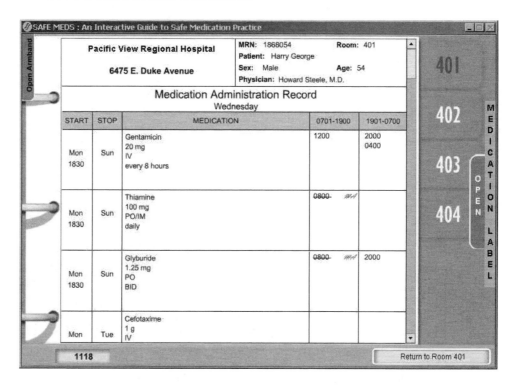

Note: The MAR changes each day. Expired MARs are stored in the patient chart.

■ VISITING A PATIENT

From the Nurses' Station, click on the room number of the patient you wish to visit in the tool bar at the bottom of your screen. Once you are inside the room, you will see a still photo of your patient in the top left corner. To verify that this is the patient you have chosen, click on the **Check Armband** icon to the right of the photo. The patient's identification data will appear. If you click on **Check Allergies** (the next icon to the right), a list of the patient's allergies (if any) will replace the photo.

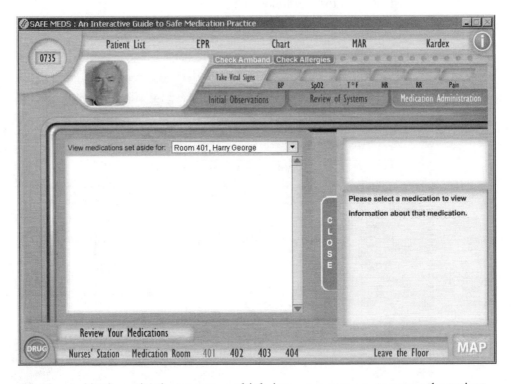

Also located in the patient's room are multiple icons you may use to assess the patient or the patient's medications. A clock is provided in the upper left corner of the room to monitor your progress in real time.

- The tool bar across the top of the screen allows you to check the **Patient List**, access the **EPR** to check or enter data, and view the patient's **Chart**, **MAR**, or **Kardex**.

- The **Take Vital Signs** icon allows you to measure up-to-the-minute blood pressure, oxygen saturation, temperature, heart rate, respiratory rate, and pain level.

- When you click on **Initial Observations**, a description appears in the text box under the patient's photo, allowing you a "look" at the patient as if you had just stepped in. To the right of this is **Clinical Alerts**, which allow you to make decisions about priority medication interventions based on emerging data collected in real time. Check this screen throughout your timed period to avoid missing critical information related to recently ordered or STAT medications.

- **Review of Systems** allows you to conduct a physical assessment of the body systems for each period of care. The summary includes the following categories of patient data:

  - Cardiovascular
  - Digestive
  - Endocrine
  - Integumentary
  - Lymphatic
  - Musculoskeletal
  - Neurologic
  - Psychosocial
  - Reproductive
  - Respiratory
  - Urologic

The data collected from these assessments can affect medication administration. For example, do you need to check an IV site before administering an intravenous medication, or evaluate a heart rhythm before administering a cardiac medication? Click on each category button for the relevant data to appear in the text box to the right of the buttons. You can exit at any time by clicking any icon on the toolbar.

- **Medication Administration** is the pathway that allows you to review and administer medications to a patient after you have prepared them in the medication room. This process is addressed further in the *How to Prepare Medications* section (pp. 20-22) and in *A Detailed Tour* (pp. 26-30).

■ HOW TO QUIT OR CHANGE PATIENTS

How to Quit: From most screens, you may click the **Leave the Floor** icon on the bottom tool bar to the right of the patient room numbers. (Note: From some screens, you will first need to click an **Exit** button or **Return to Nurses' Station** before clicking **Leave the Floor**.) When the Floor Menu appears, click **Exit** to leave the program.

How to Change Patients or Period of Care: To change patients, simply click on the new patient's room number. (You cannot receive a scorecard for a new patient, however, unless you already selected that patient on the Patient List screen.) To change to a new period of care or restart the time clock for a new patient, click the **Leave the Floor** icon and then **Restart**.

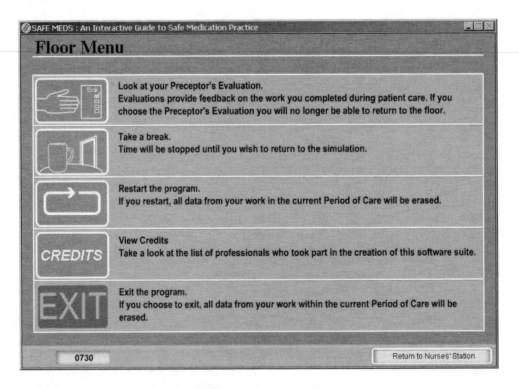

■ HOW TO PREPARE MEDICATIONS

From the Nurses' Station or the patient's room, you can access the Medication Room by clicking on the icon in the tool bar at the bottom of your screen to the left of the patient room numbers.

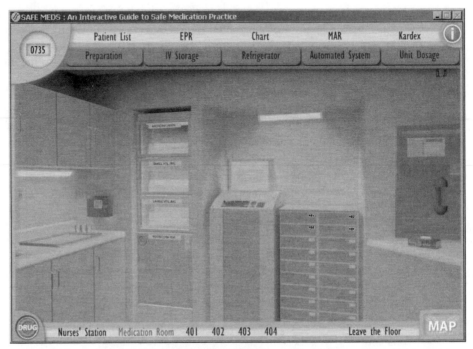

In the Medication Room you have access to the following (from left to right):

- A preparation area is located on the counter under the cabinets. To begin the medication preparation process, click on the tray on the counter or click on the **Preparation** icon at the top of the screen. The next screen leads you through a preparation sequence (called the Preparation Wizard) to prepare medications one at a time for administration to a patient. However, no medication has been selected at this time. We will do this while working with a patient in *A Detailed Tour*. To exit this screen, click on **View the Medication Room**.

- To the right of the cabinets (and above the refrigerator), IV storage bins are provided. Click on the bins themselves or on the **IV Storage** icon at the top of the screen. The bins are labeled **Microinfusion**, **Small Volume**, and **Large Volume**. Click on an individual bin to see a list of its contents. No medications are available in the bins at this time, but if they were, you could click on an individual medication and its label would appear to the right under the patient's name. Next, you would click **Put Medication on Tray**. If you ever change your mind or choose the incorrect medication, you can **Put Medication in Bin**. Click **Close Bin** in the right bottom corner to exit. **View Medication Room** brings you back to a full view of the entire room.

- A refrigerator is located under the IV storage bins to hold any medications that must be stored below room temperature. Click on it to remove your medications; then click **Close Door**. You can also access this area by clicking the **Refrigerator** icon at the top of the screen.

- To prepare controlled substances, click the **Automated System** icon at the top of the screen or click the computer monitor located to the right of the IV storage bins. A log-in screen will appear; your name and password are automatically filled in. Click **Login**. Select a patient to log medications out for; then select the drawer you wish to open. Click **Open Drawer**, choose **Put Medication on Tray**, and then click **Close Drawer**.

- Next to the Automated System is a set of drawers identified by patient room number. To access these, click on the drawers themselves or on the **Unit Dosage** icon at the top of the screen. This provides a close-up view of the drawers. Click on the room number of the patient you are working with to open that drawer. Next, click on the medication you would like to prepare for the patient, and a label appears to the right under the patient's name, listing strength, units, and dosage per unit. You can **Open** and **Close** this medication label by clicking the appropriate icon. To exit, click **Close Drawer**; then click **View Medication Room**.

At any time, you can learn about a medication you wish to prepare for a patient by clicking on the **Drug** icon in the bottom left corner of the medication room screen or by clicking the **Drug Guide** book on the counter to the right of the unit dosage drawers. The **Drug Guide** provides information about the medications commonly included in nursing drug handbooks. Nutritional supplements and maintenance intravenous fluid preparations are not included.

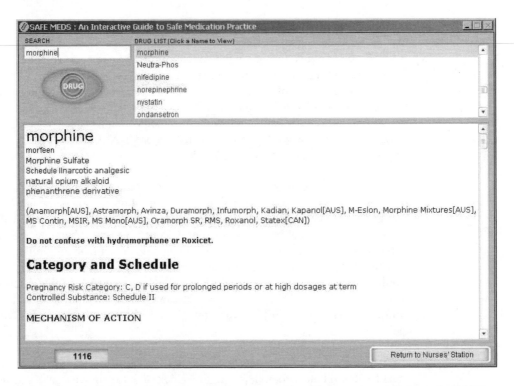

To access the MAR to review the medications ordered for a patient, click on the **MAR** icon located in the tool bar at the top of your screen. You may also click the **Review MAR** icon in the tool bar at the bottom of your screen from inside each medication storage area.

After you have chosen and prepared your medications, return to the patient's room to administer them by clicking on the room number in the bottom tool bar. Click on **Medication Administration** and follow the administration sequence.

■ PRECEPTOR'S EVALUATIONS

When you have finished a session, click on **Leave the Floor** to go to the Floor Menu. At this point, you can click on the icon next to **Look at your Preceptor's Evaluation** to receive a scorecard that provides feedback on the work you completed during patient care.

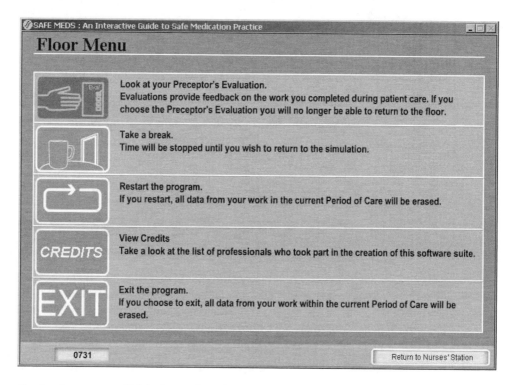

Evaluations are available for each patient you signed in for. Click on any of the **Medication Scorecard** icons to see an example. The scorecard compares the medications you administered to a patient during a period of care with what should have been administered. Table A lists the correct medications. Table B lists any medications that were administered incorrectly.

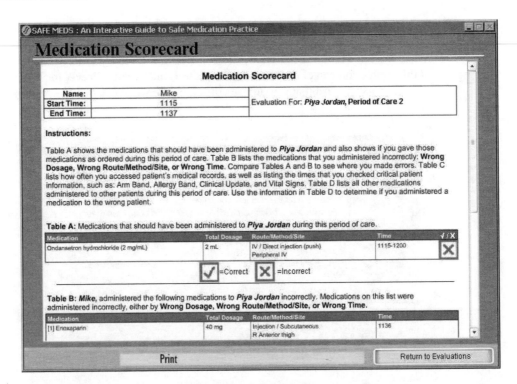

Not every medication listed on the MAR should be given. For example, a patient might have an allergy to a drug that was ordered, or a medication might have been improperly transcribed to the MAR. Predetermined medication "errors" embedded within the program challenge you to exercise critical thinking skills and professional judgment when deciding to administer a medication, just as you would in a real hospital. Use all your resources at hand, such as the patient's chart in addition to the MAR, to make your decision.

Table C lists the resources that were available to assist you in medication administration, and it documents whether and when you accessed these resources. For example, did you check the patient armband or perform a check of vital signs? If so, when?

You can click **Print** to get a copy of this report if needed. Click **Return to Evaluations** when finished.

■ FLOOR MAP

To get a general sense of your location within the hospital, click on the **Map** icon found in the lower right corner of most of the screens in the *Safe Meds* program. A floor map will appear, showing the layout of the floor you are currently on, as well as a directory of the patients and services on that floor. As you move your cursor over the directory list, the location of each room is highlighted (and vice versa). The floor map can be accessed from the Nurses' Station, Medication Room, and each patient's room.

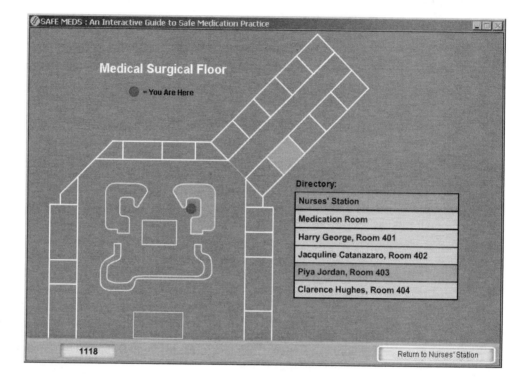

A DETAILED TOUR

If you wish to more thouroughly understand the capabilities of *Safe Meds: An Interactive Guide to Medication Administration*, take a detailed tour by completing the following section. During this tour, we will work with a specific patient to introduce you to all the different components and learning opportunities available within the software.

■ WORKING WITH A PATIENT

Sign in and select the Medical-Surgical floor for Period of Care 1 (0730-0815). On the Patient List, select Piya Jordan in Room 403; however, do not go to the Nurses' Station yet.

■ REPORT

In hospitals, when one shift ends and another begins, the outgoing nurse who attended a patient will give a verbal and sometimes a written summary of that patient's condition to the incoming nurse who will assume care for the patient. This summary is called a report and is an important source of data to provide an overview of a patient. Your first task is to get clinical report on Piya Jordan. To do this, click **Get Report** in the far right column in this patient's row. From this summary, identify the problems and areas of concern that you will need to address for this patient. When you are finished, click **Go to Nurses' Station**.

■ CHARTS

You can access the patient's chart from the Nurses' Station or from the patient's room (403). We will access it from the Nurses' Station: Click on the chart rack or on the **Chart** icon in the tool bar at the top of your screen. Next, click on chart **403** to open the medical record for Piya Jordan. Click on the **Emergency Department** tab to view a record of why this patient was admitted.

You should also click on **Surgical Reports** to learn what procedures were performed and when. Finally, review the **Nursing Admission** and **History and Physical** tabs to view information on the health history of this patient. When you are done looking at the chart, click **Return to Nurses' Station**.

■ MEDICATIONS

Open the Medication Administration Record (MAR) by clicking on the **MAR** icon in the tool bar at the top of your screen. Remember: The MAR automatically opens to the first occupied room number on the floor (in this case, Room 401, Harry George). Since you need to access Piya Jordan's MAR, click on tab **403** (her room number). Always make sure you are giving the Right Drug to the Right Patient!

Examine the list of medications prescribed for Piya Jordan. Write down the medications that need to be given during this period of care (0730-0815). For each medication, note the dosage, route, and time in the chart on the following page.

Time	Medication	Dosage	Route
0800	Digoxin	0.125 mg	IV

Click on **Return to Nurses' Station**. Next, click on **403** on the bottom tool bar and verify that you are indeed in Piya Jordan's room. Check Clinical Alerts (by clicking on **Initial Observations**) for any emerging data that might affect your medication administration priorities. Go to the patient's chart (click on the **Chart** icon; then click on **403**). When the chart has opened, click on **Physician's Orders**.

Review the orders. Have any new medications been ordered? Return to the MAR (click **Return to Room 403**; then click **MAR**). Verify that the new medications have been correctly transcribed to the MAR. Mistakes are sometimes made in the transcription process in the hospital setting, and it is sound practice to double-check any new order.

Are there any patient assessments that you will need to perform before administering these medications? If so, return to Room 403 and click on **Review of Systems** to complete those before proceeding. (Hint: Check apical pulse.)

Now click on the **Medication Room** icon in the tool bar at the bottom of your screen to locate and prepare the medications for Piya Jordan.

In the Medication Room, you must access the medications for Piya Jordan from the dispensing system in which each medication is stored. Locate each medication that needs to be given in this time period and click on **Put medication on tray** as appropriate. (Hint: Look in Unit Dosage drawer first.) When you are finished, click on **Close Drawer** and then on **View Medication Room**. Now click on the medication tray on the counter on the left side of the medication room screen to begin preparing the medications you have selected. (Note: Instead of clicking on the tray, you can click **Preparation** at top of screen.)

In the preparation area, move down the list of medications one at a time, and click **Prepare**. Follow the Preparation Wizard as directed. As an example, let's follow the preparation process for digoxin, one of the medications due to be administered to Piya Jordan during this period of care:

  Amount of medication in the ampule: 2 mL
  Enter the amount of medication you will draw up into a syringe: **0.5** mL
  Click **Next**.
  Select the patient you wish to set aside the medication for:
  Click **Room 403, Piya Jordan**.
  Click **Finish**.
  Click **Return to Medication Room**.

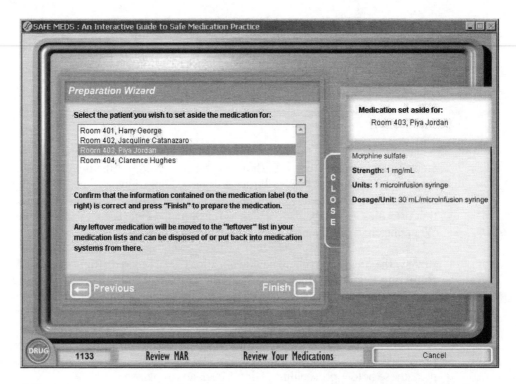

Follow the same process for the other medications due to be administered to Piya Jordan during this period of care. (Hint: Look in **IV Storage** and **Automated System**.)

■ PREPARATION WIZARD EXCEPTIONS

- Some medications in *Safe Meds* are pre-prepared by the pharmacy (e.g., IV antibiotics) and taken to the patient room as a whole. This is common practice in most hospitals.
- Blood products are not administered by students through the *Safe Meds* simulation since blood administration follows specific protocols not covered in this program.
- The *Safe Med* simulations do not allow for mixing more than one type of medication, such as regular and Lente insulins in the same syringe. In the clinical setting, when multiple types of insulin are ordered for a patient, the regular insulin is drawn up first, followed by the longer-acting insulin. Insulin is always administered in a special Unit-marked syringe.

Return to Room 403 (click on **403** on bottom tool bar).

At any time you can perform further review of systems, take vital signs, check information contained within the chart, or verify patient identity and allergies. Vital signs are often considered the traditional signs of life and include body temperature, heart rate, respiratory rate, blood pressure, oxygen saturation of the blood, and the patient's experience of pain. Inside Piya Jordan's room, click **Take Vital Signs**. These findings change over time to reflect the temporal changes you would find in a patient similar to Piya Jordan.

When you have gathered all the data you need, click **Medication Administration**. After reviewing your medications, follow the steps below.

Let's continue the process with the digoxin ordered for Piya Jordan. In the list of medications set aside for this patient, find digoxin. Under **Select**, choose **Administer**. This will bring up the Administration Wizard. Complete the Wizard sequence as follows:

- Route: **IV**
- Method: **Direct Injection**
- Site: **Peripheral IV**
- Click **Administer to Patient** arrow.
- Would you like to document this administration in the MAR? **Yes**
- Click **Finish** arrow.

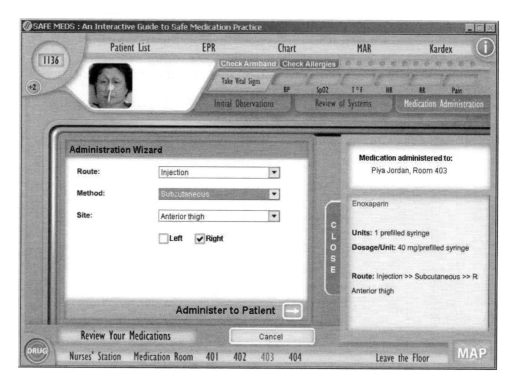

Selections are recorded by a tracking system and evaluated on a Medication Scorecard stored under Preceptor's Evaluations. This scorecard can be viewed, printed, and given to your instructor. To access the Preceptor's Evaluations, click on **Leave the Floor**. When the Floor Menu appears, click on the icon next to **Look at your Preceptor's Evaluation**. From the list of evaluations, click on **Medication Scorecard** inside the box with Piya Jordan's name.

■ **MEDICATION SCORECARD**

- First, look at Table A. Was digoxin given correctly? Did you give the other medications as ordered?
- Table B shows you which medications were given incorrectly.
- Table C addresses the resources used for Piya Jordan. Did you access the patient's chart, MAR, EPR, or Kardex as needed to make safe medication administration decisions?
- Was the patient's armband checked to verify identity? Did you check whether your patient had any known allergies to medications? Were vital signs taken?

Safe medication administration practice depends on an accurate and thorough assessment of the patient and knowledge of the medication being administered. This exercise was designed to walk you through a patient simulation in order to become familiar with the components of *Safe Meds: An Interactive Guide to Safe Medication Practice*. Your workbook will continue to lead you as you practice your skills in safe medication administration and develop both the creativity and the systematic approach needed to become a nurse who can deliver the highest quality care to all patients.

LESSON 1

Introduction

There is an alarming rise in the number of medical errors being made in the health care field. You see it in the media as major law suits come to light for errors made in hospitals as well as in outpatient settings. Medical mistakes can range from a prescription being filled with the wrong medication to surgical interventions resulting in the amputation of the wrong limb.

One of the greatest responsibilities you will have as a nurse is administering medications. The number of errors made in medication administration is also rising at a staggering rate.

> *Between 44,000 and 98,000 hospitalized Americans die as a result of medical errors each year—more than die from motor vehicle accidents, breast cancer, or AIDS.**

The purpose of this workbook is to help you understand how medication errors occur and to help you avoid making them. You will be presented with Case Scenarios, which are actual medication errors that have been made. These are discussed here to help you learn from the mistakes that have been made in nursing practice.

KEEPING YOUR PATIENTS SAFE

Our patients enter the health care setting with the expectation of receiving safe care, and yet the number of medical errors that compromise their safety is rising at an alarming rate! A patient receiving the wrong medication can be the deadliest of errors . . .. So, what exactly is a *medication error*?

> *A medication error is any preventable event in which a patient fails to receive a medication as intended by the prescriber.*

*Institute of Medicine: *To err is human: building a safer health system*, Washington, DC, 2000, National Academy Press.

31

Multiple people are involved in the chain of events that takes place from the time the order for medication is written until the patient's medication is actually administered. A medication error can occur at any point in this "drug therapy chain."

At many facilities secretaries copy orders from the order sheet onto the medication Kardex. A Kardex or Medication Administration Record (MAR) is a list of a particular patient's medications, which the nurse uses to administer the patient's medications. Many hospital secretaries are not trained in medical and pharmaceutical terminology. **It is the responsibility of the nurse to see that all orders have been checked and transcribed correctly.** Physicians (or medical students, residents, nurse practitioners, or physician assistants) write orders. We will collectively refer to anyone writing the medication order, in this context, as the prescriber.

The **prescriber** who is writing the medication order is the first link in the drug therapy chain. The written order is one of the weakest links in the chain. A blaring mistake that often happens and involves *multiple deadly* errors can occur when **insulin** is being prescribed. A prescriber might write a "U" instead of writing out the word "units." The "U," when written quickly, can appear as a "0." Because this mistaken "0" comes directly after the number of units, this can result in the dose given to be *ten times the intended dose*. Schools of medicine are addressing this with medical students to minimize this particular error, and the Joint Commission on Accreditation of Healthcare Organizations (JCAHO) is attempting to limit this mistake by discontinuing "U" from its acceptable abbreviations. But it still happens. There is also the problem of legibility in the orders. As the nurse verifying the order—*DO NOT HESITATE TO CLARIFY THE ORDER*. If you are uncomfortable for *any* reason, call the prescriber and tell him or her your concerns. Your patient's life may depend on it.

Another problem in the written order is that of "naked decimals." When a medication order includes a decimal, the physician needs to write a "0" before the decimal (digoxin 0.5 mg). Without the "0" the decimal point may be missed (a naked decimal), resulting in a medication error of multiple proportions. The physician, however, should *not* write a "0" *after the decimal point* (5.0). This can also lead to deadly mistakes if the decimal is missed.

It is also the nurse's responsibility to be sure that the dosage that is ordered is a safe dosage for the patient.

Case Scenarios

A physician ordered morphine .5 mg IV for a 9-month-old baby. The secretary missed the decimal and transcribed the order onto the MAR as morphine 5 mg IV. An inexperienced nurse followed the directions on the MAR and gave the baby 5 mg of morphine IV, and the baby died. This is an example of "death by decimal."

Bottom line . . . if you are not comfortable with a medication order . . . question it!

The next link in the drug therapy chain is the **pharmacist.** Consider the pharmacist to be the ultimate resource regarding medication safety. Remember, however, that medication errors can occur at any link in the chain. For example, a patient was to receive lomustine (an antineoplastic drug) to treat brain cancer. It is typically given "1 dose every 6 weeks." The prescriber ordered it to be given at bedtime ("hs"). However, the patient received it *every* night ("*q*hs") for 9 nights and died. For 9 consecutive days, the pharmacist sent the medication to be administered—a human error. There are also pharmacy technicians who stock the unit dose drawers or bins. The covering licensed pharmacist is responsible for all actions within the pharmacy but is not checking everything the technicians are doing on a daily basis. Pharmacists and pharmacy technicians are human, and they make errors.

The next link in the chain is the **nurse**. Administering medications will be your biggest responsibility as a practicing nurse. **You are legally responsible for all of the medications you give.** You need to know *what* you are giving. You need to know that what you are giving is safe for your patient. If you are not comfortable and confident with a medication order, you need to first clarify it with the prescriber, and second, check with a drug reference guide to determine that what is ordered by the prescriber and delivered by the pharmacist is truly safe to administer. If you are still not sure the drug is an appropriate drug and dose for your patient, don't give the medication. The nurse needs to be the patient's "safeguard."

If in doubt—don't hand out.

Check with the prescriber immediately.

CLARIFY THE DRUG ORDER AND KNOW WHAT YOU ARE GIVING IS SAFE

As the nurse administering a medication, you need to know what you are giving and what it is prescribed for. You need to know that the dose ordered is a *safe* dose. You need to know that the drug is not contraindicated for your patient when given with the patient's other drugs. You need to review what adverse effects you will be monitoring. AND you need to know any nursing consideration, especially what you need to do before you give the drug. (Does the patient need an apical pulse checked before receiving digoxin?) All hospital units should be equipped with drug reference books so that the nurse can research any drug that is not familiar.

This is a great deal of information to check for each drug you give. But, once you learn to check the apical/radial pulse with digoxin, you won't need to check the drug reference each time you give it. You will incorporate this safety check into your everyday practice.

Drug reference books give you very important information. Most have drug compatibility charts so that you know when giving an IV medication whether it is compatible with medications that may be in the primary IV or in the tubing left from the last mini-bag that was hung.

What if the drug you are giving is not listed in the drug guide on your unit? Your institution should be replacing outdated drug guides with the latest editions, but there still may be occasions when you can't find the information you need. Your next best reference would be your hospital pharmacist. The pharmacist should be able to fax you any information you need. Another reference is the Internet. Most drugs (even the newest ones) will have information you can research on the Internet. If you still can't verify that this medication is safe for this patient . . . don't give it. *If in doubt—don't hand out.*

Pacific View Regional Hospital	MRN: 1868057	Room: 502
	Patient: Delores Gallegos	
6475 E. Duke Avenue	Sex: Female	Age: 82
	Physician: Gerald Moher, M.D.	

Physician's Orders

Weight: 160 lbs   **Age:** 82

Day/Time	Orders	Signature
Mon 1400	**Order Type:** General	*Gerald Moher, M.D.*
	1. Admit to Skilled Nursing Unit, Internal Medicine Service.	
	2. Activity: Up ad lib.	
	3. Diet: Regular, low salt pending Dietary consult recommendations.	
	4. Dietary consult.	
	5. Skin care TID to rash.	
	6. Intake and Output every 8 hours.	
	7. Vital signs every 8 hours.	
	8. Labs: Basic metabolic panel every other day to include sodium, potassium, chloride, CO_2, blood urea nitrogen, glucose, creatinine.	
	9. Furosemide 40 mg PO daily.	
	10. Captopril 12.5 mg PO TID.	
	11. Metoprolol 25 mg PO daily.	
	12. Docusate sodium 100 mg PO daily.	
	13. Bisacodyl 10 mg daily prn no bowel movement per rectum.	
	14. Daily weight.	

Exercise 1

 You will be going to Pacific View Regional Hospital to administer medications for your assigned patient. Please remember when administering medications to all patients:

√ Check the MAR against the physician's order to be sure that all orders have been transcribed correctly.
√ Document all medications after the patient has received them.

> **Assignment:** Administer medications to Delores Gallegos, Room 502. Floor: Skilled Nursing. Period of Care 1: 0730–0815.

 1. List the medications ordered for your patient to receive during the current time period from the Physician's Orders.

2. Do any of these orders contain decimals? If the decimal is "missed" when the order is transcribed, what dosage will actually be administered?

3. When you compare what the prescriber ordered with the medications listed on the MAR, do you find any discrepancies?

4. *Critical Thinking:* What is your safest nursing action based on your findings in question 2?

METRIC SYSTEM

In the world of medication administration, the metric system is used for weights and measures. As the nurse responsible for administering medications, you need to understand the metric system.

You can memorize conversion tables and easily learn the math involved in converting mcg to mg. But you need to *understand* the difference between *weight* and *volume*.

Drug dosages will be **ordered** by weight (*grams*, milli*grams*, micro*grams*) but will be **administered** by volume (milli*liters*).

For example, the prescriber orders morphine elixir *10 mg* po q4h for pain, and the morphine elixir comes from the pharmacy as morphine *10 mg in 5 mL*. You will need to administer the *5 mL* of solution. It is imperative that you understand the difference between the dosage (10 mg) and the volume (5 mL).

Case Scenarios

A premature infant in a neonatal ICU was receiving aminophylline (bronchodilator). Instead of administering the 7.4 mg that was ordered, the nurse administered 7.4 mL, which was 185 mg. The baby developed tachycardia and other signs of theophylline toxicity and died.

The nurse administered volume instead of dosage.

The Current Teaching Strategy

THE FIVE "RIGHTS" OF MEDICATION ADMINISTRATION

Patient safety has to be the top priority of all nurses practicing in today's health care environment. Nursing students have long been taught that administering medications according to the five "rights" will ensure that patients will be kept safe. The five "rights" are:

1. Right Patient
2. Right Drug
3. Right Dose
4. Right Route
5. Right Time

Some textbooks have added a sixth:

6. Right Documentation

Some have added a seventh:

7. Patient Right to Refuse

Some are now up to ten:

8. Right Assessment
9. Right Patient Education
10. Right Evaluation

For practicing nurses, as well as student nurses, this enlarging laundry list is truly overwhelming. How many of us can remember all of the rights and whether we've included each one? Is there any wonder that students are getting confused and that practicing nurses are making errors? And to top it off, even after covering all ten rights, there are still some safety issues missing. What if the patient has an allergy to the medication? What if someone already gave the medication? These are issues not covered by "the rights," be it five, seven, or ten of them. There is a better way—a new strategy for safe medication administration.

37

A New Strategy—Three Valid Checks and Three Bedside A's

To incorporate safety into medication administration, you must validate *three separate times* that you actually have in your hand the drug that the prescriber ordered for this time. With the MAR in front of you, you need to perform three *valid* checks with the labeled medication:

1. When you take the medication out of the patient's drawer
2. As you pour the medication (or put the labeled package in a medication cup)
3. At the bedside, administering the drug

This is not a lengthy process, but it multiplies the safety potential. Take a look at a sample medication order and when you would be validating the order with the medication label:

The MAR reads, "*digoxin 0.25 mg po qd. It is due at 8:00 a.m. and has not yet been signed as given.*"

Be sure to check the MAR order completely, including all of the information above. This valid check will include the drug name, dose, route, frequency, time, and whether or not it has already been given. By doing these three checks, you are validating all of this information. It's not a matter of remembering what information to check. It's all right there on the MAR. Just read the order and follow across the page to see if it's yet been documented as "given."

Also check that each medication you are giving is not an expired medication. Check the expiration date on each drug.

Check All of This Information on the MAR

1st Check:

Take the medication out of the right patient's drawer (verifying that the name and room number on the drawer match the name and room number on the MAR), and look at the medication label. Read the MAR: "*digoxin 0.25 mg po qd. It is due at 8:00 a.m. and has not yet been signed as given.*" Check on the label that you really have digoxin 0.25 mg per tablet. If the label does not match the MAR, this is the point where you may need to do a math calculation. Check the expiration date on the medication label. If the label and the MAR match, move to your second check.

2nd Check:

As you pour the medication (or place the unopened pack in a medication cup), look at the MAR and read: "*digoxin 0.25 mg po qd. It is due at 8:00 a.m. and has not yet been signed as given.*" Look at the medication label, checking that you really have digoxin 0.25 mg per tablet. If you're giving multiple medications, do your second check and place unopened pills in a medication cup. That way, if the patient refuses the medication, or it needs to be held, you will know which pill to hold.

3rd Check:

> The MAR reads, "*digoxin 0.25 mg po qd. It is due at 8:00 a.m. and has not yet been signed as given*." Check this information against the label before opening the package at the bedside.

You have now completed three valid checks.

It sounds time-consuming, but once you have incorporated these steps, it becomes very easy and much safer.

When you proceed to the bedside to administer the medications, **take the MAR with you**. Once you get to the bedside, it is very important to check that you are administering medication to the correct patient and that you are keeping him or her safe. An easy way to remember the steps you need to do at the bedside is to remember the "Three A's":

1. **Armband**—Identify the patient by checking his armband against the name and patient ID number on the MAR. You may feel silly if this is a patient you know well, but when administering medications to multiple patients, this is an area of "high error potential." It is extremely easy when you are busy to give a patient someone else's medications.

2. **Allergies**—When you have determined that you have the correct patient by identifying the armband, you must next determine whether the patient has any medication allergies. Many institutions have a second ID bracelet that lists medication allergies. When checking the ID band, also check for an allergy band. Ask the patient about any medication allergies. Again, if this is a patient you know well, he or she may say, "I haven't developed any allergies since you gave me my pills yesterday!" It's better to recheck each time than to administer a medication that causes an allergic reaction.

3. **Assessments**—With many medications, assessments need to be made *prior* to administering a medication. For example, with the digoxin on which you performed your three valid checks, the patient needs an apical pulse reading before administration of the medication. If the pulse is less than 60 beats or greater than 110 beats per minute, the medication is routinely held. If administering a pain medication, assess an accurate pain level to determine later whether the pain medication is effectively relieving the patient's pain. These types of assessments are crucial to patient safety.

Remember "3's"

Three Valid Checks

1. As you take the medication out of the drawer
2. As you pour the medication
3. Before opening the package at the bedside

The Three Bedside "A's"

1. Armband
2. Allergies
3. Assessments

It is much easier to remember groups of three like this than to remember five rights (or ten).

It is also important to listen to the patient. It's very easy to get caught up in work to stay on schedule, but one of your most valuable resources is the patient. **Tell the patient what medications you are giving.** If patients tell you they don't take a pill for their blood pressure, listen to them. This is a definite "red flag" to the nurse that this could be the wrong medication or the wrong patient. Don't just blindly administer a medication that the patient questions.

Once the patient has received all medications, *immediately* document the medications given. This prevents a duplication error. If you fail to document, another nurse may administer the medication a second time. Immediate documentation is a very important safety factor.

Case Scenarios

A nurse was giving medications to the same group of patients for the third night in a row. After giving sleeping pills to two male patients in the same room, the nurse was leaving the room when she heard one patient say to the other, "Gee, last night my sleeping pill was orange." And the other patient responded, "Yeah, last night mine was pink." The nurse had confused the two patients and administered the wrong medication to each.

Which of the Three Bedside "A's" did the nurse miss?

The Road to Medication Safety—Putting the Strategies Together

We've covered a lot of information, so let's put all of the pieces together.

Strategies to Reduce Medication Errors:

1. Verify that each medication on the MAR has been checked against the physician's order.
2. Clarify any inconsistencies.
3. If unfamiliar with a medication, look up the medication in a drug book. Be sure to check that the dose is safe, and check the nursing considerations (*What do I need to do before I can administer this drug?*).
4. With the MAR in hand, check the complete label three times:
   - When you take the medication out of the drawer
   - When you pour the medication (or place the package in a medication cup)
   - At the bedside before administering the medication

5. Perform any needed medication calculation, and verify the calculation with a second nurse.
6. Perform the Three Bedside A's:
   - Armband
   - Allergies
   - Assessments
7. Explain what medications you are giving.
8. Listen to your patients. If they have concerns, they are probably justified. **Listen to them.**
9. If you are uncomfortable giving a medication, **don't give it**.
   If in doubt—don't hand out.
10. After all medications have been administered, immediately document the medications given.

Pacific View Regional Hospital 6475 E. Duke Avenue	MRN: 1868092 Room: 403 Patient: Piya Jordan Sex: Female Age: 68 Physician: Steven Joffe, M.D.

Physician's Orders

Weight:	Age:	
Day/Time	**Orders**	**Signature**
Wed 0730	**Order Type:** General 1. Discontinue Meperidine PCA. 2. Change PCA to Morphine sulfate 1 mg/mL. 1 mg every 10 min, 4-hour lockout 24 mg. No loading dose. 3. Discontinue Promethazine. 4. Ondansetron 4 mg IV every 6 hours prn nausea. 5. Insert saline lock and administer 2 units packed red blood cells IV transfusion. 6. Enoxaprin 40 mg subQ every 12 hours to start this evening. 7. Potassium chloride 20 mEq IV in 250 mL NS to infuse over 2 hours.	*Howard Steele, M.D.*

Pacific View Regional Hospital 6475 E. Duke Avenue	MRN: 1868092 Room: 403
	Patient: Piya Jordan
	Sex: Female Age: 68
	Physician: Steven Joffe, M.D.

Physician's Orders

Weight: **Age:**

Day/Time	Orders	Signature
Tue 1900	**Order Type:** Postoperative 1. Admit to Medical Surgical Unit. 2. Vital signs every 4 hours. 3. Intake and Output every 8 hours. 4. Diet: NPO. 5. Daily weight. 6. Activity: Out of bed to chair in morning. 7. Telemetry monitoring. 8. Oxygen 2L by nasal cannula. 9. Incentive spirometer 10 times per hour while awake. 10. Nasogastric tube to low continuous suction. 11. Foley to gravity drainage. 12. Jackson-Pratt drain at incision site to bulb suction. 13. Sequential compression device to lower extremities. 14. IV D5NS with 20mEq KCl/L at 100 mL/hr. 15. Cefotetan 1 g IV q12h x 6 doses. 16. Meperidine PCA 25 mg loading dose; 10 mg/mL every 10 min; 4 hour lockout 240 mg.	*James Rudnick, M.D.*
		cont. next page

Pacific View Regional Hospital 6475 E. Duke Avenue	MRN: 1868092 Room: 403 Patient: Piya Jordan Sex: Female Age: 68 Physician: Steven Joffe, M.D.

Physician's Orders *(cont.)*		

Weight: **Age:**

Day/Time	Orders	Signature
Tue 1900	**Order Type:** Postoperative 17. Digoxin 0.125 mg IV daily to start Wednesday morning. 18. Famotidine 20 mg IV q12h. 19. Promethazine 12.5-25 mg IV q4-6h prn nausea. 20. Acetaminophen 650 mg per rectum q6h prn fever >102 F. 21. Labs Wednesday: Hemoglobin and hematocrit. Chem 7. PT/INR. Digoxin level.	*James Rudnick, M.D*

EXERCISE 1

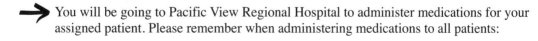

You will be going to Pacific View Regional Hospital to administer medications for your assigned patient. Please remember when administering medications to all patients:

√ Check the MAR against the physician's order to be sure that all orders have been transcribed correctly.
√ Perform three valid checks on each medication.
√ Perform the Three Bedside A's (armband, allergies, assessments).
√ Document all medications after the patient has received them.

Assignment: You have been assigned to administer medications to Piya Jordan, Room 403. Floor: Medical-Surgical. Period of Care 1: 0730–0815.

1. List the medications ordered for the patient to receive during the current time period, including prn medications.

2. Open the patient's unit dosage medication drawer. Pull up each medication listed. Compare the medications in the drawer "on hand" with what the doctor ordered. Clarify any inconsistencies.

3. Prepare the medications to be given. Proceed to the patient's bedside to administer the medications. What specific assessments (the third Bedside A) need to be performed with these specific medications?

4. *Critical Thinking:* The patient is to receive cefotetan IV. When performing the Bedside A's, did you note any drug allergies for this patient? Is it safe to administer this IV antibiotic to this patient? Why? What are the potential adverse effects of this medication?

Proceed to Period of Care 2: 1115–1200.

    5. Review physician's orders for acetaminophen. Proceed to the bedside and review the vital signs. Should the patient receive this medication? Why or why not? What is the discrepancy?

ROUTES OF ADMINISTRATION

Oral Route

The nurse needs to assess the patient who is receiving oral medications (po). If the patient has dysphasia (difficulty swallowing), the oral medication may need to be administered in a liquid form. The prescriber will need to change the order to an alternate route. There are, however, certain medications that may be crushed and mixed with pudding or other soft foods to aid the patient in swallowing the medication. *Sustained-release (or delayed-release) tablets cannot be crushed or the capsule opened.*

When giving po liquid medication, the liquid is sometimes dispensed with a syringe, and the syringe tip is placed in the patient's mouth, and the medication is slowly inserted until the patient is able to swallow. Use of a syringe makes measuring medication more accurate. *However, medication errors have been made when nurses inject the liquid oral medication into an IV or central line.*

Case Scenarios

A nurse was giving digoxin elixir po to a patient. When the medication came from the pharmacy, it was supplied in a syringe for accurate dosing. Instead of administering the dose orally, the nurse connected the syringe to the patient's intravenous lock and injected the liquid intravenously. The patient died.

Pacific View Regional Hospital	MRN: 1868051	Room: 503
	Patient: Kathryn Doyle	
6475 E. Duke Avenue	Sex: Female	Age: 79
	Physician: Gerald Moher, M.D.	

Physician's Orders

Weight: 105 lbs	**Age:** 79	

Day/Time	Orders	Signature
Mon 1000	**Order Type:** Transfer	*Gerald Moher, M.D.*
	1. Admit to Skilled Nursing Unit, Internal Medicine.	
	2. Diet: Regular, soft mechanical.	
	3. Vital signs every 8 hours.	
	4. Activity: Ambulate at least four times a day. Patient needs to get up to use bathroom.	
	5. Physical therapy to direct rehabilitation.	
	6. Dietary consult.	
	7. Social work consult.	
	8. Calcium citrate 2 tablets PO BID.	
	9. Ferrous sulfate 325 mg PO TID with meals.	
	10. Docusate sodium 100 mg PO daily.	
	11. Ibuprofen 600 mg PO TID.	
	12. Oxycodone 2.5 mg with acetaminophen 325 mg 1 or 2 tablets PO every 4-6 hours prn for pain.	
	13. Acetaminophen 325-650 mg PO every 4 hours prn for mild pain or fever >101.5 F.	
	14. Daily weight.	

EXERCISE 2

 You will be going to Pacific View Regional Hospital to administer medications for your assigned patient. Please remember when administering medications to all patients:

√ Check the MAR against the physician's order to be sure that all orders have been transcribed correctly.
√ Perform three valid checks on each medication.
√ Perform the Three Bedside A's (armband, allergies, assessments).
√ Document all medications after the patient has received them.

Assignment: You have been assigned to administer medications to Kathryn Doyle, Room 503. Floor: Skilled Nursing. Period of Care 1: 0730–0815.

 1. List the medications ordered for the patient to receive during the current time period. Look up each of the po medications to be given in the Drug Guide provided on the counter in the Nurses' Station or in the Medication Room. Note the classification, safe dose, and any nursing implications or contraindications.

2. You have read in the report that the patient is complaining of difficulty swallowing. The patient is requesting that all oral medications be crushed and administered in applesauce. Is this a safe alternative for the medications noted above?

3. What is the safest nursing action based on your findings in question 2?

	MRN: 1868015	Room: 501
Pacific View Regional Hospital	Patient: William Jefferson	
	Sex: Male	Age: 75
6475 E. Duke Avenue	Physician: Marlene Dirkson, M.D.	

Physician's Orders

Weight: 183 lbs   **Age:** 75

Day/Time	Orders	Signature
Sun 1100	**Order Type:** Transfer	*Marlene Dirkson, M.D*
	1. Admit to Skilled Nursing Unit.	
	2. Request old charts to floor.	
	3. Diet: 1800 K calorie, no added salt; include snacks midmorning, midafternoon, and bedtime in 1800 calorie total.	
	4. Intake and Output every 8 hours.	
	5. Vital signs every 8 hours. Notify physician if T >100 F; BP >180 systolic, <120 systolic, >98 diastolic.	
	6. Up as tolerated.	
	7. Occupational therapy consult/treatment plan for ADL functioning.	
	8. Physical therapy consult/treatment plan for strengthening, home exercise program.	
	9. Hydrochlorothiazide 50 mg PO daily.	
	10. Metformin 850 mg PO BID.	
	11. Rosiglitazone 8 mg PO daily.	
	12. Enalapril 10 mg PO daily.	
	13. Atenolol 25 mg PO daily	
		cont. next page

Pacific View Regional Hospital 6475 E. Duke Avenue	MRN: 1868015 Room: 501 Patient: William Jefferson Sex: Male Age: 75 Physician: Marlene Dirkson, M.D.

Physician's Orders *(cont.)*

Weight: 183 lbs   **Age:** 75

Day/Time	Orders	Signature
Sun 1100	**Order Type:** Transfer 14. Rivastigmine 4.5 mg PO BID. 15. Ibuprofen 400 mg PO at bedtime and every 4 hours prn pain 16. Ciprofloxacin 500 mg PO every 12 hours for 14 days. 17. Bowel program: Milk of Magnesia 30 mL PO prn if no bowel movement for 3 days. 18. Finger-stick daily before lunch. Notify physician if blood sugar >180. 19. WBC with differential, Hgb, Hct, fasting blood glucose Monday morning.	*Marlene Dirkson, M.D*

 Next, proceed to Room 501, William Jefferson. Floor: Skilled Nursing. Period of Care 1: 0730–0815.

Review the medications in the patient's drawer. Locate the liquid (elixir) form of the medication rivastigmine.

 4. What is the drug's concentration? (How many mg per mL?)

5. What is the physician's order for this medication? Compare this order with the patient's MAR.

6. How many mL will you administer?

7. *Critical Thinking:* Look at the enalapril drug order. Which medication, also in the patient's drawer, has a similar name and dosage? Is the patient currently receiving that medication too? What is the safest nursing action?

Injectable Route

Many medications are administered by injection. The dose will be ordered by weight (units, grams, milligrams, micrograms) but will be administered by volume (milliliters).

For example: The patient is receiving morphine sulfate 5 mg IM q4h for pain. If the vial comes with a label that reads *Morphine Sulfate 10 mg/mL*, you will need to perform a calculation. You will then need to administer 0.5 mL, which equals 5 mg.

An exception to this general rule is insulin. Insulin is ordered in units and ***always*** administered in units in an insulin syringe.

You may be giving an injection by one of several routes:
- Intradermal
- Subcutaneous (subQ)
- IM (Intramuscular)
- Z-track (also an intramuscular)
- IV (intravenous)

Special information related to each injectable route:

- **Intradermal injections** are given just below the surface of the skin into the dermis layer. This type of injection is used in allergy testing and tuberculin skin tests. The nurse does not apply pressure to the intradermal injection site because the medication is quickly absorbed. *1-mL syringe with 26- to 28-gauge needle— 1/2-inch needle. Usually 0.1 mL of solution.*

- **Subcutaneous injections** (subQ) are given into the fatty layer of subcutaneous tissue. To access the subcutaneous layer, the skin should be pinched, the needle inserted, and the skin released. Once the skin is released, the medication is then administered. The skin may be massaged after the injection, unless the medication administered is an anticoagulant like heparin. Massaging a heparin injection may increase risk for bruising because of its anticoagulant effect. Heparin should be administered into the abdomen, 1–2 inches from the umbilicus (laterally or below). *1- to 3-mL syringe with 25- to 29-gauge needle—1/2- to 5/8-inch needle. Usually 0.5 to 1 mL of solution.*

- **Intramuscular injections** (IM) are given deep into the muscle. The nurse needs to accurately assess a proper intramuscular site to avoid injury to the patient, such as trauma to the bones, blood vessels, or nerves. The skin is generally spread taut during an IM injection to gain access to deep muscle. Most IM injections need to be aspirated to ensure muscle injection and not injection into a vein. If you aspirate and find a blood return, discard the medication and start the injection process over. *2- to 3-mL syringe with 21- to 23-gauge needle—1.5- to 3-inch needle. Usually 0.5 to 2 mL of solution.*

- **Z-track** is a type of intramuscular injection that is used for medications that are irritating to tissue. When preparing for the injection, pull the skin to one side of the site. Inject the medication, and aspirate for blood; if there is no blood, inject the medication, leave the needle in place for 10 seconds, and then release the skin. This creates a zigzag track that prevents the irritating medication from leaking into the tissue.

Intravenous Route

Intravenous injections (IV medications) are medications that can be administered via the intravenous route for rapid infusion, for large doses, and for patients who cannot tolerate po medications. They are given by either peripheral IV or central venous catheters. There are complications associated with this route of administration, including infection and too rapid infusion, which can lead to shock and death. IV medications can be:
1. Diluted in the primary IV bag.
2. Piggyback—secondary small-volume IV infusion.
3. IV push.

This must be specified by the physician's order. It is important for the nurse to assess the IV site prior to injection and to infuse the medication at the correct rate to avoid the complications mentioned above.

Case Scenarios

A physician ordered a concentrated liquid medication to be given SL (sublingually). It was misinterpreted by the nurse to be given SL (saline lock). The concentrated po liquid was given IV push.

Pacific View Regional Hospital 6475 E. Duke Avenue	MRN: 1868011 Room: 404 Patient: Clarence Hughes Sex: Male Age: 73 Physician: Thomas Price, M.D.

Physician's Orders

Weight: 207 lbs   **Age:** 73

Day/Time	Orders	Signature
Tue 0600	**Order Type:** General 1. Discontinue Foley catheter this morning, may straight cath every 6-8 hours if unable to void. 2. Discontinue cryocuff. 3. Change dressing every day and prn. 4. Activity: Up to chair twice a day. Physical therapy to ambulate. 5. Discontinue IV infusion; convert to a saline lock. 6. Discontinue Morphine PCA. 7. Discontinue Cefazolin after 6th dose. 8. Oxycodone with acetaminophen 1-2 tablets PO every 4-6 9. Labs: Hemoglobin, hematocrit and prothrombin tomorrow morning.	*Thomas Price, M.D.*

Pacific View Regional Hospital	MRN: 1868011	Room: 404
	Patient: Clarence Hughes	
6475 E. Duke Avenue	Sex: Male	Age: 73
	Physician: Thomas Price, M.D.	

Physician's Orders

Weight: 207 lbs   **Age:** 73

Day/Time	Orders	Signature
Mon 0715	**Order Type:** General	*Myron Kuhn, M.D.*

1. Monitor vital signs and circulation, motion, and sensation every 8 hours.

2. Wean off oxygen with oxygen saturation greater than 90% on room air.

3. Continuous passive motion (CPM) machine 6 hours per day to L knee with the following goals:
   45 degrees postop day 1
   60 degrees postop day 2
   75 degrees postop day 3
   90 degrees postop day 4
   Notify MD if unable to meet goals as specified.

4. Patient to be out of CPM at night; L leg should be flat with pillow under the heel.

5. Activity: Up in chair today before noon. Physical therapy to ambulate this afternoon.

6. Decrease IV infusion to 30 mL/hr if patient is taking adequate oral fluids.

7. Enoxaparin 30 mg subQ every 12 hours to start this evening.

8. Labs: Hemoglobin, hematocrit, and prothrombin tomorrow morning.

Pacific View Regional Hospital 6475 E. Duke Avenue	MRN: 1868011	Room: 404
	Patient: Clarence Hughes	
	Sex: Male	Age: 73
	Physician: Thomas Price, M.D.	

Physician's Orders

Weight: 207 lbs   **Age:** 73

Day/Time	Orders	Signature
Sun 1600	**Order Type:** Postoperative 1. Admit to the Medical Surgical floor--diagnosis status post left total knee arthroplasty. 2. Diet: Clear liquids tonight; advance to regular diet as tolerated. 3. Vital signs every 4 hours including circulation, motion and sensation checks. 4. Intake and Output measurement every 8 hours. 5. Oxygen 2L flow by nasal cannula. 6. Incentive spirometer 10 times every hour while awake. 7. Activity: Bedrest. 8. Foley catheter to gravity drainage. 9. Wound drain--hemovac to compression suction. 10. Reinforce dressing to L knee as needed. 11. Cryocuff to left knee. Sequential compression device to R leg while in bed. 12. IV D5.45 NS with 20 mEq KCl per liter to infuse at 125 mL/hr. 13. Cefazolin 2 grams IV every 8 hours X 6 doses. 14. Morphine sulfate IV PCA 1 mg every 10 minutes/lock out 24 mg every 4 hours.	*Thomas Price, M.D.* cont. next page

Pacific View Regional Hospital	MRN: 1868011	Room: 404
	Patient: Clarence Hughes	
6475 E. Duke Avenue	Sex: Male	Age: 73
	Physician: Thomas Price, M.D.	

Physician's Orders *(cont.)*

Weight: 207 lbs   **Age:** 73

Day/Time	Orders	Signature
Sun 1600	**Order Type:** Postoperative	*Thomas Price, M.D.*
	15. Docusate sodium 100 mg PO BID.	
	16. Celecoxib 100 mg PO BID.	
	17. Timolol maleate 0.25% ophthalmic solution 2 drops to both eyes every 12 hours.	
	18. Pilocarpine 1% ophthalmic solution 2 drops to both eyes every 12 hours.	
	19. Promethazine 12.5 to 25 mg IV every 6 hours prn for nausea.	
	20. Aluminum hydroxide with magnesium and simethicone 30 mL PO every 8 hours prn for gastrointestinal upset.	
	21. Bisacodyl 10 mg suppository per rectum every 12 hours	
	22. Milk of magnesia 30 mL PO every 8 hours pm for constipation.	
	23. Acetaminophen 325-650 mg PO every 4-6 hours prn for fever >101 F.	
	24. Temazepam 15 mg PO at bedtime prn for sleep.	
	25. Labs: Hemoglobin and hematocrit in morning.	

EXERCISE 3

 You will be going to Pacific View Regional Hospital to administer medications for your assigned patient. Please remember when administering medications to all patients:

√ Check the MAR against the physician's order to be sure that all orders have been transcribed correctly.
√ Perform three valid checks on each medication.
√ Perform the Three Bedside A's (armband, allergies, assessments).
√ Document all medications after the patient has received them.

Assignment: You have been assigned to administer medications to Clarence Hughes, Room 404. Floor: Medical-Surgical. Period of Care 1: 0730–0815.

 1. List the medications ordered for the patient to receive during the current time period, including prn medications. In the Drug Guide provided, look up each drug's classification and safe dose range.

2. One of the medications ordered for your patient is enoxaparin 30 mg subQ. Prepare this medication and perform your three valid checks, making sure that you have the correct amount of the medication in the prefilled syringe.

3. When administering this medication, which site will you choose? How do you determine the appropriate site?

4. What assessments need to made for the patient receiving this medication? Which laboratory test will you be monitoring for this patient because he is receiving enoxaparin?

5. *Critical Thinking:* This patient is complaining of pain. Which medication is ordered for pain? Open the automated dispensing machine and remove the pain medication. How many doses are available? What is your safest nursing action?

Pacific View Regional Hospital	MRN: 1868018	Room: 302
	Patient: Tommy Douglas	
6475 E. Duke Avenue	Sex: Male	Age: 6
	Physician: Robert Gardner, M.D.	

Physician's Orders

Weight:	Age: 6	
Day/Time	**Orders**	**Signature**
Mon 0700	**Order Type:** General	*Robert Gardner, M.D.*
	1. Normal saline 200 mL IV bolus x 1 now.	
	2. Lidocaine 2% solution 0.5 mL instilled into endotracheal tube prior to suctioning.	
	3. Increase IMV to 25.	

Pacific View Regional Hospital 6475 E. Duke Avenue	MRN: 1868018 Room: 302 Patient: Tommy Douglas Sex: Male Age: 6 Physician: Robert Gardner, M.D.

Physician's Orders

Weight:	Age: 6

Day/Time	Orders	Signature
Wed 0600	**Order Type:** Transfer 1. Transfer to Telemetry Unit. 2. Diagnosis: Traumatic Brain Injury, status post ventriculostomy placement. Condition: Critical. 3. Neurosurgery/neurology, Social services, Pastoral services, and Child life specialist to follow. 4. Vital signs: Every hour. 5. Continuous cardiac monitor (heart rate 80-160). 6. Continuous pulse oximetry (alarms 92-100). 7. Dopamine 1200 mg/100 mL NS (1 mL = 10 mcg/kg/min) at 20 mcg/kg/min or 2 mL/hour IV. 8. Artificial tears, drops as needed to both eyes every 4 hours. 9. Norepinephrine 12 mg/100 mL NS (1 mL = 0.1 mcg/kg/min) at 1 mL/hour. 10. Cefazolin 500 mg IV every 6 hours. 11. D5.45 NS at 55 mL/hr. 12. Normal saline with Heparin 1 unit/mL to radial arterial line at 3 mL/hr.	*Robert Gardner, M.D.*

Pacific View Regional Hospital **6475 E. Duke Avenue**	**MRN:** 1868018 **Room:** 302 **Patient:** Tommy Douglas **Sex:** Male **Age:** 6 **Physician:** Robert Gardner, M.D.	

Physician's Orders

Weight:	**Age:** 6	

Day/Time	Orders	Signature
Mon 2100	**Order Type:** General 1. Acetaminophen 200 mg via nasogastric tube every 4 hours prn temperature >101.5 F. 2. Artificial tears with drops as needed to both eyes every 4 hours.	*Robert Gardner, M.D.*

→ Next you are assigned to care for Tommy Douglas, Room 302. Floor: Pediatrics. Period of Care 2: 1115–1200.

 6. List the medications ordered for this patient. List all of the various "routes" ordered.

7. "Lidocaine 0.5 mL/ETT before suctioning" is ordered for this patient. If you are unfamiliar with this route, how will you clarify this? What is the safest nursing action? What is the purpose for this medication?

Pacific View Regional Hospital	MRN: 1868092	Room: 403
	Patient: Piya Jordan	
6475 E. Duke Avenue	Sex: Female	Age: 68
	Physician: Steven Joffe, M.D.	

Physician's Orders

Weight:	Age:	
Day/Time	**Orders**	**Signature**
Wed 0730	**Order Type:** General	*Howard Steele, M.D.*

Order Type: General

1. Discontinue Meperidine PCA.

2. Change PCA to Morphine sulfate 1 mg/mL. 1 mg every 10 min, 4-hour lockout 24 mg. No loading dose.

3. Discontinue Promethazine.

4. Ondansetron 4 mg IV every 6 hours prn nausea.

5. Insert saline lock and administer 2 units packed red blood cells IV transfusion.

6. Enoxaprin 40 mg subQ every 12 hours to start this evening.

7. Potassium chloride 20 mEq IV in 250 mL NS to infuse over 2 hours.

Pacific View Regional Hospital	**MRN:** 1868092	**Room:** 403
	Patient: Piya Jordan	
6475 E. Duke Avenue	**Sex:** Female	**Age:** 68
	Physician: Steven Joffe, M.D.	

Physician's Orders

Weight: **Age:**

Day/Time	Orders	Signature
Tue 1900	**Order Type:** Postoperative	*James Rudnick, M.D.*
	1. Admit to Medical Surgical Unit.	
	2. Vital signs every 4 hours.	
	3. Intake and Output every 8 hours.	
	4. Diet: NPO.	
	5. Daily weight.	
	6. Activity: Out of bed to chair in morning.	
	7. Telemetry monitoring.	
	8. Oxygen 2L by nasal cannula.	
	9. Incentive spirometer 10 times per hour while awake.	
	10. Nasogastric tube to low continuous suction.	
	11. Foley to gravity drainage.	
	12. Jackson-Pratt drain at incision site to bulb suction.	
	13. Sequential compression device to lower extremities.	
	14. IV D5NS with 20mEq KCl/L at 100 mL/hr.	
	15. Cefotetan 1 g IV q12h x 6 doses.	
	16. Meperidine PCA 25 mg loading dose; 10 mg/mL every 10 min; 4 hour lockout 240 mg.	
		cont. next page

Pacific View Regional Hospital 6475 E. Duke Avenue	MRN: 1868092	Room: 403
	Patient: Piya Jordan	
	Sex: Female	Age: 68
	Physician: Steven Joffe, M.D.	

Physician's Orders *(cont.)*

Weight:	Age:	

Day/Time	Orders	Signature
Tue 1900	**Order Type:** Postoperative 17. Digoxin 0.125 mg IV daily to start Wednesday morning. 18. Famotidine 20 mg IV q12h. 19. Promethazine 12.5-25 mg IV q4-6h prn nausea. 20. Acetaminophen 650 mg per rectum q6h prn fever >102 F. 21. Labs Wednesday: Hemoglobin and hematocrit. Chem 7. PT/INR. Digoxin level.	*James Rudnick, M.D.*

 Next proceed to Room 403, Piya Jordan. Floor: Medical-Surgical. Period of Care 1: 0730–0815.

 8. List the IV medications this patient is currently receiving.

9. The patient is receiving digoxin IV. How many mg are ordered? How many mg per mL in vial? How many mL will you administer? Perform calculations. What bedside assessment must be performed prior to administration?

10. *Critical Thinking:* The patient has an order for potassium chloride 20 mEq per 250 mL NS over 2 hours. (Be sure to check the STAT/PRE-OP/ONE TIME section of the MAR.) When hanging this medication by piggyback, what happens to the main IV? Calculate total IV fluid for this shift.

Special Issues With Pediatric Doses

An area of concern regarding medication errors is that involved with pediatric drug doses. Because of the variations in patient size and weight, the "standard" drug doses prescribed for the adult patient would often result in an *overdose* for the pediatric patient.

Therefore, the pediatric dose is often ordered by "dose by weight" for the pediatric patient. The prescriber may order a certain amount of *micrograms* or *milligrams* per *kilogram* of body weight. This will, therefore, require the nurse to accurately calculate the drug dose.

The nurse will need to calculate two factors in determining the correct drug dose:

- Converting pounds to kilograms
- Calculating the amount of drug to be administered according to the determined weight

Once the dose is calculated, it is advised that any drug ordered in this format be checked by a second nurse before it is administered.

Dangers in Automated Infusion Pumps

Infusion pumps were introduced to the health care setting in the 1960s to deliver specific amounts of medications intravenously within a specific time range. Medication is mixed into an IV bag, and the pump delivers a certain amount of the fluid to the patient as programmed by the health care provider. Over the past 40 years, safety features of the infusion pumps have improved dramatically. However, if a health care facility is using outdated machines, there is a danger of "free flow." When the IV tubing is removed from the pump, fluid and the medications it contains have the possibility of running rapidly into the patient. This has been the cause of numbers of medication-related deaths over the years.

Case Scenarios

A patient who had undergone surgery for a ruptured abdominal aortic aneurysm was started on nitroprusside sodium to lower blood pressure via the IV pump. Only a few milliliters of the drug were needed, but during transport from the Recovery Room to the ICU, the patient went into shock. At some point during transfer, the tubing had been removed from the pump without the gravity clamp being engaged. The patient died from "free flow" of the medication.

Pacific View Regional Hospital 6475 E. Duke Avenue	MRN: 1868018	Room: 302
	Patient: Tommy Douglas	
	Sex: Male	Age: 6
	Physician: Robert Gardner, M.D.	

Physician's Orders

Weight:	Age: 6	

Day/Time	Orders	Signature
Wed 0600	**Order Type:** Transfer	*Robert Gardner, M.D.*

Order Type: Transfer

1. Transfer to Telemetry Unit.

2. Diagnosis: Traumatic Brain Injury, status post ventriculostomy placement.
   Condition: Critical.

3. Neurosurgery/neurology, Social services, Pastoral services, and Child life specialist to follow.

4. Vital signs: Every hour.

5. Continuous cardiac monitor (heart rate 80-160).

6. Continuous pulse oximetry (alarms 92-100).

7. Dopamine 1200 mg/100 mL NS (1 mL = 10 mcg/kg/min) at 20 mcg/kg/min or 2 mL/hour IV.

8. Artificial tears, drops as needed to both eyes every 4 hours.

9. Norepinephrine 12 mg/100 mL NS (1 mL = 0.1 mcg/kg/min) at 1 mL/hour.

10. Cefazolin 500 mg IV every 6 hours.

11. D5.45 NS at 55 mL/hr.

12. Normal saline with Heparin 1 unit/mL to radial arterial line at 3 mL/hr.

EXERCISE 4

 You will be going to Pacific View Regional Hospital to administer medications for your assigned patient. Please remember when administering medications to all patients:

√ Check the MAR against the physician's order to be sure that all orders have been transcribed correctly.
√ Perform three valid checks on each medication.
√ Perform the Three Bedside A's (armband, allergies, assessments).
√ Document all medications after the patient has received them.

Assignment: You have been assigned to administer medications to Tommy Douglas, Room 302. Floor: Pediatrics. Period of Care 1: 0730–0815.

 1. List the drugs that are ordered by weight.

2. How much does this patient weigh? Convert the weight from kilograms to pounds. Show your work.

3. For norepinephrine, how many micrograms are ordered? Set up the calculation needed to determine the correct number of mL you need to administer to set your pump at the correct mL/hr.

 Sign out and return to Period of Care 3: 1500–1545.

4. This rate is now increased to 0.3 mcg/kg/hr. Recalculate the dose to administer via pump at mL/hr.

Pacific View Regional Hospital 6475 E. Duke Avenue	MRN: 1868082 Room: 301 Patient: George Gonzalez Sex: Male Age: 11 Physician: Robert Gardner, M.D.

Physician's Orders

Weight:	Age: 11 years	
Day/Time	**Orders**	**Signature**
Tue 2200	**Order Type:** General	*Robert Gardner, M.D.*
	1. Admit to the Pediatric Unit.	
	2. VS every 4-6 hours.	
	3. Weigh Wednesday morning.	
	4. Urinalysis and pH Wednesday morning.	
	5. Check blood sugars pre-meals, at bedtime, and at 0200.	
	6. Notify physician for blood sugar less than 80 or greater than 250.	
	7. Give 12 Units NPH insulin + 6 Units Lispro insulin subQ prebreakfast.	
	8. Give 8 Units NPH insulin + 4 Units Lispro insulin subQ predinner.	
	9. 2200-calorie ADA diet, 3 meals, 3 snacks.	
	10. Psychiatric and nutrition consults.	
	11. May saline lock IV when IV infusion completed. Flush with 3-5 mL Normal Saline every 8 hours prn.	
	12. Initiate discharge planning and diabetic re-education.	

Sign out and proceed to Room 301, George Gonzalez. Floor: Pediatrics. Period of Care 1: 0730–0815.

5. List the types and amounts of insulin ordered for this patient.

6. *Critical Thinking:* If you need to administer two different types of insulin, describe the procedure for mixing two types of insulin in the same syringe. Which site will you choose to administer this insulin? Why?

Administration of Medications to the Older Adult

Another group of patients with special concerns when administering medications is the elderly population. With aging comes multiple physiological changes that increase the risk for making a medication error. With increased age comes increased health concerns, and elderly patients are often taking multiple medications, which may interact with one another, producing unwanted side effects. With age there is a general "slowdown" in bodily functions, making metabolism and excretion of drugs slower. This can cause too much of the drug to be in a patient's system and increase the likelihood of an overdose.

Elderly patients may also have compliance issues. With failing memories, they may not remember to take a medication, or they may have taken it but don't recall and so take it again. The expense of medications is another compliance issue. For patients who must choose between food and medication, they may not be *able* to take the prescribed medication.

Teaching is an essential component in nursing care, and educating the elderly in safe medication administration is a must. Making sure that patients are physically able to take their medications is crucial—they may need to request "nonchildproof" medication lids. Keeping their medications in a safe area, out of children's reach, and away from any harmful sources is also very important. Using large print in any medication directions will also help to safeguard against taking the wrong medication.

All of these areas will help the patient be safe and reduce the risk for medication errors in the elderly.

Case Scenarios

An elderly woman was discharged home from the hospital with eye drops to be instilled. She was later brought to the ER with her eyelids glued shut. She had stored the eye drops in a cupboard next to the superglue and had instilled the superglue into her eyes in error.

Pacific View Regional Hospital **6475 E. Duke Avenue**	**MRN:** 1868015 **Room:** 501 **Patient:** William Jefferson **Sex:** Male **Age:** 75 **Physician:** Marlene Dirkson, M.D.

Physician's Orders

Weight: 183 lbs   **Age:** 75

Day/Time	Orders	Signature
Sun 1100	**Order Type:** Transfer 1. Admit to Skilled Nursing Unit. 2. Request old charts to floor. 3. Diet: 1800 K calorie, no added salt; include snacks midmorning, midafternoon, and bedtime in 1800 calorie total. 4. Intake and Output every 8 hours. 5. Vital signs every 8 hours. Notify physician if T >100 F; BP >180 systolic, <120 systolic, >98 diastolic. 6. Up as tolerated. 7. Occupational therapy consult/treatment plan for ADL functioning. 8. Physical therapy consult/treatment plan for strengthening, home exercise program. 9. Hydrochlorothiazide 50 mg PO daily. 10. Metformin 850 mg PO BID. 11. Rosiglitazone 8 mg PO daily. 12. Enalapril 10 mg PO daily. 13. Atenolol 25 mg PO daily	*Marlene Dirkson, M.D.* **cont. next page**

Pacific View Regional Hospital 6475 E. Duke Avenue	**MRN:** 1868015 **Room:** 501 **Patient:** William Jefferson **Sex:** Male **Age:** 75 **Physician:** Marlene Dirkson, M.D.

Physician's Orders *(cont.)*

Weight: 183 lbs   **Age:** 75

Day/Time	Orders	Signature
Sun 1100	**Order Type:** Transfer 14. Rivastigmine 4.5 mg PO BID. 15. Ibuprofen 400 mg PO at bedtime and every 4 hours prn pain 16. Ciprofloxacin 500 mg PO every 12 hours for 14 days. 17. Bowel program: Milk of Magnesia 30 mL PO prn if no bowel movement for 3 days. 18. Finger-stick daily before lunch. Notify physician if blood sugar >180. 19. WBC with differential, Hgb, Hct, fasting blood glucose Monday morning.	*Marlene Dirkson, M.D.*

EXERCISE 5

 You will be going to Pacific View Regional Hospital to administer medications for the assigned patient. Please remember when administering medications to all patients:

√ Check the MAR against the physician's order to be sure that all orders have been transcribed correctly.
√ Perform three valid checks on each medication.
√ Perform the Three Bedside A's (armband, allergies, assessments).
√ Document all medications after the patient has received them.

Assignment: You have been assigned to administer medications to William Jefferson, Room 501. Floor: Skilled Nursing. Period of Care 1: 0730–0815.

1. Look at the MAR. Write down the drug name, safe dose, and nursing implications for the antihypertensive drugs. Use the Drug Guide found in the Medication Room or the Nurses' Station.

2. Look up *enalapril* in the Drug Guide. Is the dosage ordered for this patient a safe dose? What assessments will you make before administering this drug?

3. Look up *hydrochlorothiazide* in the Drug Guide. Is the dosage ordered for this patient a safe dose? What is this drug given for?

4. Look up *atenolol* in the Drug Guide. What is this drug given for?

5. *Critical Thinking:* Do you have any concerns related to the medications ordered for this patient? What side effects might this patient experience from these medications that could affect his safety? What is your safest nursing action?

→ Restart the program and go to Period of Care 2: 1115–1200.

6. *Critical Thinking:* The patient is receiving ciprofloxacin 500 mg po every 12 hours. What lab values are important for this patient, related to this particular medication?

The Nervous System

NEUROLOGICAL ASSESSMENTS

Depending on a patient's diagnosis, the nurse may need to assess neurological function. This is done by assessing the level of consciousness (LOC), the reaction of pupils to light, and the strength of the extremities. All of these assessments give the nurse a baseline of neurological function, and frequent reassessment helps determine critical changes that may occur.

ASSESSMENTS FOR PAIN MEDICATION

Pain is whatever degree of "hurt" the patient describes it to be. It is of utmost importance that the nurse realizes that the patient's pain is real and is whatever the patient reports.

Pain assessment, often called the fifth vital sign, is important, and the nurse needs to be aware of a patient's pain level to determine the effectiveness of the pain medications a patient is receiving. The nurse needs to ask the patient to "rate" pain on a pain scale. If "1" is minimal pain, and "10" is the worst pain ever experienced, the nurse can determine the rate of pain. If the patient is a "9" and after receiving pain medication only comes down to an "8," the pain medication may need to be reevaluated.

PAIN MEDICATIONS

Medications to combat pain, or "analgesics," may be narcotic (opioid) or nonnarcotic (nonopioid).

1. Nonopioid Analgesics

   These are the first choice for treatment of mild to moderate pain and include:

   - NSAIDS (nonsteroidal antiinflammatory)
   - Acetaminophen

75

They act on the peripheral nervous system at the pain receptor sites. They prevent the formation of prostaglandins in inflamed tissue. In this way the pain receptors are not stimulated.

NSAIDS—This group of drugs includes aspirin and ibuprofen and works to relieve pain, reduce inflammation, and reduce fever. Aspirin should not be used in children under 12 years of age because of the risk for Reye's syndrome. This group of drugs may relieve mild to moderate pain. Side effects include gastric disturbance, renal failure, and bleeding. These drugs should be taken with food to minimize gastric disturbance.

Acetaminophen (Tylenol)—Acetaminophen is given to relieve pain and reduce fever but does not have an antiinflammatory effect. It can enhance the use of narcotic analgesics. Side effects include liver damage, especially if taken in large quantities or if taken with alcohol (maximum dose is 4 grams in 24 hours).

2. Opioid Analgesics

Narcotic analgesics act on the central nervous system and not only relieve moderate to severe pain but also suppress respirations and cough centers in the medulla of the brainstem.

Morphine—A potent narcotic analgesic. Morphine may be taken orally, IM, subQ, or IV route. Morphine works by depressing the central nervous system and therefore depresses respirations. Patients receiving morphine need frequent assessment of respirations.

Codeine—Effective narcotic analgesic given po or IM, subQ. Codeine can be given with acetaminophen for pain relief. Codeine has an antitussive effect and also causes respiratory depression.

Many of these medications also cause constipation.

Special Considerations for Controlled Substances

Opioid analgesics have the disadvantage of tolerance, physical dependence, and addiction. It is very important, however, that the nurse does not classify a patient in pain as "drug-seeking." Nurses need to assess a patient's pain by what the patient says, not by history or demeanor.

VERBAL AND TELEPHONE ORDERS

We have seen that the prescriber's written order is the first link in the drug therapy chain and is often the cause for medication errors. Illegible handwriting, use of multiple abbreviations, and look-alike drug names are examples of problems that can lead to the failure of a patient receiving the intended medication.

In some cases prescribers may verbally order a medication, either in person, as in the case of an emergency, or by telephone, when they are not readily available to write a drug order. The nurse can write the physician's order, and then the prescriber will verify that order with a signature when he or she becomes available. This method of ordering medications has its own unique set of problems that can lead to a medication error. There is a phenomenon known as "confirmation bias," where people will associate a drug name that is most familiar to them. This is also a problem when the written order is not available. Nurses may write what they *think* they heard, but this may not always be accurate. Without the order in writing, there is no way to "double-check" what the physician intended.

As a nurse receiving a verbal order, especially a telephone order, you should ask the physician to repeat the medication name and dose, spell the drug name, and ask what the reason is for the medication. This validation would greatly reduce the risk for a medication error being made.

Case Scenarios

An emergency room physician gave a verbal order for morphine 2 mg IV. The nurse heard morphine 10 mg IV. The nurse gave the patient 10 mg of morphine, and the patient experienced a respiratory arrest.

Pacific View Regional Hospital 6475 E. Duke Avenue	MRN: 1868015	Room: 501
	Patient: William Jefferson	
	Sex: Male	Age: 75
	Physician: Marlene Dirkson, M.D.	

Physician's Orders

Weight: 183 lbs   **Age:** 75

Day/Time	Orders	Signature
Sun 1100	**Order Type:** Transfer	*Marlene Dirkson, M.D*
	1. Admit to Skilled Nursing Unit.	
	2. Request old charts to floor.	
	3. Diet: 1800 K calorie, no added salt; include snacks midmorning, midafternoon, and bedtime in 1800 calorie total.	
	4. Intake and Output every 8 hours.	
	5. Vital signs every 8 hours. Notify physician if T >100 F; BP >180 systolic, <120 systolic, >98 diastolic.	
	6. Up as tolerated.	
	7. Occupational therapy consult/treatment plan for ADL functioning.	
	8. Physical therapy consult/treatment plan for strengthening, home exercise program.	
	9. Hydrochlorothiazide 50 mg PO daily.	
	10. Metformin 850 mg PO BID.	
	11. Rosiglitazone 8 mg PO daily.	
	12. Enalapril 10 mg PO daily.	
	13. Atenolol 25 mg PO daily	
		cont. next page

Pacific View Regional Hospital 6475 E. Duke Avenue	MRN: 1868015 Room: 501 Patient: William Jefferson Sex: Male Age: 75 Physician: Marlene Dirkson, M.D.

Physician's Orders (cont.)

Weight: 183 lbs   **Age:** 75

Day/Time	Orders	Signature
Sun 1100	**Order Type:** Transfer 14. Rivastigmine 4.5 mg PO BID. 15. Ibuprofen 400 mg PO at bedtime and every 4 hours prn pain 16. Ciprofloxacin 500 mg PO every 12 hours for 14 days. 17. Bowel program: Milk of Magnesia 30 mL PO prn if no bowel movement for 3 days. 18. Finger-stick daily before lunch. Notify physician if blood sugar >180. 19. WBC with differential, Hgb, Hct, fasting blood glucose Monday morning.	*Marlene Dirkson, M.D*

EXERCISE 1

 You will be going to Pacific View Regional Hospital to administer medications for your assigned patient. Please remember when administering medications to all patients:

√ Check the MAR against the physician's order to be sure that all orders have been transcribed correctly.
√ Perform three valid checks on each medication.
√ Perform the Three Bedside A's (armband, allergies, assessments).
√ Document all medications after the patient has received them.

Assignment: You have been assigned to administer medications to William Jefferson, Room 501. Floor: Skilled Nursing. Period of Care 1: 0730–0815.

 1. List the medications ordered for your patient to receive during the current time period.

2. When you checked the physician's orders with the MAR, did you note any discrepancies?

3. Prepare the patient's medications and proceed to the bedside. Perform the Three Bedside A's. What assessments will you include for the medications you are administering?

Pacific View Regional Hospital 6475 E. Duke Avenue	**MRN:** 1868054 **Room:** 401 **Patient:** Harry George **Sex:** Male **Age:** 54 **Physician:** Howard Steele, M.D.

Physician's Orders

Weight: 143 lbs   **Age:** 54

Day/Time	Orders	Signature

Tue 0800	**Order Type:** General
	
	1. Change Cefotaxime to Ceftazidime 2 g IV every 8 hours.
	
	2. Clean left foot wound with Normal saline, wipe dry with sterile gauze, then apply occlusive dressing to open area three times a day.
	
	3. Please have physical therapist evaluate patient.
	
	4. New lab orders today:
	    Folic acid level.
	    Repeat CBC and electrolytes.
	    Amylase and lipase.
	    Schedule bone scan of left
	    foot for today.
		Howard Steele, M.D.

Pacific View Regional Hospital 6475 E. Duke Avenue	MRN: 1868054	Room: 401
	Patient: Harry George	
	Sex: Male	Age: 54
	Physician: Howard Steele, M.D.	

Physician's Orders

Weight: 145 lbs   **Age:** 54

Day/Time	Orders	Signature
Mon 1830	**Order Type:** General	*Howard Steele, M.D.*
	1. Admit to Medical Unit.	
	2. Vital signs every 4 hours.	
	3. Send culture and sensitivity of wound if not done in ED.	
	4. Blood cultures from two different sites if T >102 F.	
	5. Foley catheter to gravity drainage.	
	6. Activity: Bedrest.	
	7. Keep left foot elevated on two pillows.	
	8. Have Wound Care Team evaluate left foot wound.	
	9. Do dressing changes per Wound Care Team orders.	
	10. IV of Normal saline at 125 mL/hr.	
	11. Continue Cefotaxime 1 g every 6 hours (started in ED).	
	12. Gentamicin 20 mg IV every 8 hours. Draw peak and trough with 5th dose.	
	13. Chlordiazepoxide hydrochloride 50 mg IV every 4-6 hours prn agitation.	
	14. Thiamine 100 mg PO or IM on admission and then daily.	
	15. 1800 calorie ADA diet.	

Next proceed to Room 401, Harry George. Floor: Medical-Surgical. Period of Care 1: 0730–0815. Compare the physician's order with the MAR.

 4. Open the small volume IV bin in the medication room. If you are administering this patient's cephalosporin, which one will you choose?

5. What is the danger in stocking two medications with "look-alike" names in the patient's drawer?

6. *Critical Thinking:* If you are administering the patient's gentamycin, look up this medication in the Drug Guide. What assessments will you make before hanging this medication IV? What ongoing assessment will you make?

SPECIAL MEDICATIONS FOR NEURO PATIENTS

1. Central Nervous System Stimulants

   Amphetamines—Used to treat narcolepsy, obesity, and attention deficit disorder.
   Analeptics (caffeine)—Used to treat newborn apnea, restore mental alertness.

2. Central Nervous System Depressants

   Sedatives, Hypnotics—Sedatives depress the CNS at a minimal level and are sometimes used to treat anxiety. At a higher level, these drugs are used as a hypnotic to induce sleep. At a very high level, these drugs may be used as an anesthetic.

Categories of Sedative Hypnotics:

- Barbiturates
- Benzodiazepines
- Piperdinediones

3. Narcotic Analgesics (see **Pain Medications**)

4. Muscle Relaxants

Muscle relaxants affect skeletal muscles and are used to control skeletal muscle hyperactivity and muscle spasms. Muscles spasms are involuntary muscle contractions that happen as impulses travel from the muscle to the spinal cord and back to the muscle. Skeletal muscle relaxants are believed to break this cycle by acting as a CNS depressant.

5. Anticonvulsants

Anticonvulsants suppress the abnormal electrical activity in the brain that occurs during a seizure. These drugs are given on a long-term basis and do not cure epilepsy but, rather, control the seizure activity. It requires 1 to 4 weeks to reach a therapeutic level, depending on the medication. Examples of anticonvulsant medications include:

- Phenytoin sodium (Dilantin)
- Fosphenytoin (Cerebyx)
- Tegretal
- Phenobarbital
- Neurontin

Some anticonvulsants are also used to treat pain adjunctively; e.g., Neurontin.

Case Scenarios

A 6-year-old was admitted to the ER with a skull fracture. When he developed seizures, the physician ordered Cerebyx (antiseizure) 300 mg. The vial stated, "Cerebyx 50 mg per mL." The vial contained 10 mL (a total of 500 mg), but this information was listed on a different section of the label. Instead of a total of 500 mg per vial, the nurse thought each vial contained 50 mg. The nurse, therefore, drew up and administered 6 vials (3000 mg) instead of the 300 that was ordered. The child died.

As seen with this medication error, labels sometimes prove to be less than nurse-friendly.

DRUG LABELS

Packaging and labeling designs for the pharmaceutical companies reside under a concept known as "trade dress." This is the *look* of the drug package and must be clean, neat, and tidy. The pharmaceutical company will produce a label they feel will enhance the product's marketability. If they have a product that is working well, drug companies have been resistant to make changes to the successful package, even when safety has been called into question.

An example of this occurred with the packaging of *lidocaine*. It formerly came in two strengths:

- 2% (100 mg) for IV bolus infusions
- 2 gm (2000 mg) to mix in IV solutions

Both of the syringes had a red "2" on the label. Errors occurred when the 2 gm (2000 mg) was given IV push (bolus). When these errors were reported, no changes were made to the labeling until the pharmaceutical companies were sued, and the packaging labels have since been removed from the market.*

There is also the problem of inadequate information on the label. **It is of utmost importance** that the nurse knows how many milligrams (dose) are in each milliliter (amount of fluid) and how many of these milliliters need to be given. Had the nurse known this information in the previous medication error (the 6-year-old who received an overdose of Cerebyx), this would have had a very different outcome. The fact that she needed 6 vials should have alerted the nurse to a problem.

USP/FDA Recommends Improved and Uncrowded Injection Labels, USP Quality Review, No. 62, 8/98, Rockville, MD, The United States Pharmacopeial Convention, Inc.

Pacific View Regional Hospital **6475 E. Duke Avenue**	**MRN:** 1868092	**Room:** 403
	Patient: Piya Jordan	
	Sex: Female	**Age:** 68
	Physician: Steven Joffe, M.D.	

Physician's Orders

Weight: **Age:**

Day/Time	Orders	Signature
Wed 0730	**Order Type:** General	*Howard Steele, M.D.*
	1. Discontinue Meperidine PCA.	
	2. Change PCA to Morphine sulfate 1 mg/mL. 1 mg every 10 min, 4-hour lockout 24 mg. No loading dose.	
	3. Discontinue Promethazine.	
	4. Ondansetron 4 mg IV every 6 hours prn nausea.	
	5. Insert saline lock and administer 2 units packed red blood cells IV transfusion.	
	6. Enoxaprin 40 mg subQ every 12 hours to start this evening.	
	7. Potassium chloride 20 mEq IV in 250 mL NS to infuse over 2 hours.	

EXERCISE 2

 You will be going to Pacific View Regional Hospital to administer medications for your assigned patient. Please remember when administering medications to all patients:

√ Check the MAR against the physician's order to be sure that all orders have been transcribed correctly.
√ Perform three valid checks on each medication.
√ Perform the Three Bedside A's (armband, allergies, assessments).
√ Document all medications after the patient has received them.

Assignment: You have been assigned to administer medications to Piya Jordan, Room 403. Floor: Medical-Surgical. Period of Care 2: 1115–1200.

Open the patient's medication drawer and pull up ondansetron hydrochloride:

   1. According to the drug "label," how many mg per mL?

2. How many mL are in the entire vial?

3. Check the Physician's Orders. How many mg has the prescriber ordered? How many mL will you draw up?

4. When you compared the physician's order with the MAR, were there any discrepancies? What is the safest nursing action?

5. *Critical Thinking:* Your patient is very nauseated and requests this medication (ondansetron) to be given. It has been transcribed incorrectly. What can you do to hasten correction of the problem and give the medication?

LESSON 4

The Cardiovascular System

The cardiovascular system is comprised of:

- Heart
- Blood vessels (arteries, veins, capillaries)
- Blood

The blood, rich in oxygen and nutrients, moves through the arteries, and the arteries narrow to arterioles. Capillaries transport this rich, nourished blood to body cells and absorb waste products. The deoxygenated blood is returned to circulation by the venules to the veins for elimination by the lungs and kidneys. The effectiveness of this system depends on the following:

1. The heart's ability to pump blood
2. The patency of the blood vessels
3. The quantity and quality of blood

CONGESTIVE HEART FAILURE

Congestive heart failure (CHF) is the inability of the heart to pump sufficient blood to meet the needs of the tissues for oxygen and nutrients. Congestive heart failure can be:

1. Left-sided failure—producing pulmonary edema and dyspnea.
2. Right-sided failure—producing pedal edema, ascites, hepatic congestion.
(Or it may affect both sides of the heart at the same time.)

In patients with CHF, the overworked heart cannot meet the demands placed on it, and blood is not ejected effectively from the ventricles. Because the heart cannot meet the demands, the blood supply to certain organs is reduced. The organs most dependent on blood supply, the heart and brain, are the last to be deprived of blood. The kidneys are less dependent on blood supply, so the blood may be shunted away. This results in accumulation of waste and fluid, resulting in pulmonary edema, shortness of breath, and kidney failure.

89

Signs and Symptoms of CHF

- Dyspnea on exertion
- Fatigue
- Ankle edema
- Jugular vein distention
- Cough
- Weight gain

The drug of choice for treating CHF is digoxin (Lanoxin). It works in three ways:

1. Increased myocardial contraction
2. Decreased heart rate
3. Decreased conduction of heart cells

Because of the dramatic effect digoxin has on the heart, it is vital to assess the patient's heart rate (apical heart rate for accuracy) *and* to hold the drug and notify the physician if the apical pulse is less than 60 beats or greater than 110 beats per minute. An abnormal heart rhythm for the patient on digoxin is a sign of toxicity and indicates the need to question giving the medication.

Case Scenarios

A nurse was administrating multiple medications to her 42-year-old patient. One of the medications was digoxin. When administering digoxin, the nurse needed to assess the patient's pulse rate and hold the medication if the patient's pulse rate was below 60. The nurse failed to assess the patient's pulse (the third Bedside A). The pulse was 36 beats/minute. The nurse gave the digoxin, and the patient suffered a cardiac arrest and died.

DISTRACTIONS IN PREPARATION

As described earlier, there is a "chain of events" that occurs from the time the medication order is written until the patient actually receives the medication. A medication error is *any preventable event in which a patient fails to receive a medication intended by the prescriber*. If the medication order is written correctly *and* transcribed correctly *and* filled correctly by the pharmacist, the nurse is the next link in the chain of events.

As the nurse preparing a patient's medications, concentrate on the important task at hand. In our busy world, busy schedules, and busy lifestyles, we all become accustomed to "multitasking"—doing a number of things at the same time. This **cannot apply** to the task of medication preparation. Medication preparation requires your undivided attention. Whether it's retrieving the correct drug from the automated dispensing machine or calculating the number of milliliters to deliver the correct number of milligrams, you need your maximum amount of concentration.

In order to achieve this, minimize the distractions in your workplace. You may need to take your patient's medication and MAR into the medication room or any "quiet" location to minimize distractions during medication preparation. Preparing your medications on the medication cart in the busy hallway with patients, physicians, health care providers, family members, and other nurses interrupting your process with questions, demands, and orders is *not* a safe environment. It's very easy to lose your train of thought and make a medication error. Performing three valid checks (or five patient rights), as well as dose calculations, takes concentration. An interruption in this process is an *accident waiting to happen*.

AUTOMATED MEDICATION-DISPENSING DEVICES

Acting as ATMs for medications, these ***automated medication-dispensing devices*** are part robot and part computer. Introduced in the 1980s, these machines for controlled substances are commonplace in many hospitals today, as seen in Pacific View Regional Hospital. Usually referred to by their trade name—the Pyxis, the Baxter, the Omnicell— their purpose is to save nurses time, to track medications used for accurate billing, to track what each nurse is dispensing, and to prevent patients from receiving the wrong medication. Each patient's information, including the medications ordered by the physician, is entered into the machine's memory. Each medication nurse must enter his or her code and password to gain access. He or she then chooses the particular patient and is allowed access to whatever medications *that* patient is ordered to receive. Once the medication's name is chosen, the drawer that contains that medication opens up, and the nurse can retrieve that medication, in its unit dose packet, and administer it to the patient. In theory, this practice should greatly reduce the errors, which occur at the dispensing *and* administration steps of the medication process. The disadvantage to this system occurs on large units where 30 patients all have medications due at 8:00 a.m. There can be a long line of nurses waiting to use the dispensing machine. Patients may actually have a longer wait for their medications. There is also a way for nurses to override the computer and to have access to another patient's medications and "borrow," thereby setting up the patient for an error. If the hospital units have enough machines to accommodate large numbers of patients *and* if they are used as designed, they have a potential to make medication administration a much safer procedure.

It is still the nurse's responsibility to check the medication three times for accuracy. The pharmacists and pharmacy technicians stock the dispensing units. Don't trust that just because the "Colace" drawer opens up, that it is always stocked with only Colace. Check the unit dose packet and know that you have the correct drug. Remember to perform the ***three valid checks*** on each medication.

Many hospitals have purchased or leased these dispensing machines. Most of the new models have the potential to accommodate computerized physician's orders and the "art" of bar coding medications.

BAR CODING

We have all seen the "bar code" system utilized. In the grocery store when an item is "scanned" by the cash register, it uses the item's bar code for needed information. The bar code supplies the name of the item and its price and provides information for inventory purposes. This technology is currently in use in the Veteran's Administration health care system. There are bar codes on all the nurses' ID badges, patients' ID bands, and on each unit-dose package of medication. The medication cart (an **automated medication-dispensing device**) is equipped with a hand-held scanner allowing the nurse to scan his or her ID, the patient's ID, and the medication. If the medication matches the physician's order for the medication, and it is the correct time for the drug, the computer gives a "green light," and the medication drawer opens, allowing the nurse access. The transaction is recorded in the medical record, and an error is prevented. When combined with computerized physician order entry, this could greatly reduce medication errors.

Pacific View Regional Hospital 6475 E. Duke Avenue	MRN: 1868092 Room: 403 Patient: Piya Jordan Sex: Female Age: 68 Physician: Steven Joffe, M.D.

Physician's Orders

Weight: **Age:**

Day/Time	Orders	Signature
Wed 0730	**Order Type:** General 1. Discontinue Meperidine PCA. 2. Change PCA to Morphine sulfate 1 mg/mL. 1 mg every 10 min, 4-hour lockout 24 mg. No loading dose. 3. Discontinue Promethazine. 4. Ondansetron 4 mg IV every 6 hours prn nausea. 5. Insert saline lock and administer 2 units packed red blood cells IV transfusion. 6. Enoxaprin 40 mg subQ every 12 hours to start this evening. 7. Potassium chloride 20 mEq IV in 250 mL NS to infuse over 2 hours.	*Howard Steele, M.D.*

EXERCISE 1

 You will be going to Pacific View Regional Hospital to administer medications for your assigned patient. Please remember when administering medications to all patients:

√ Check the MAR against the physician's order to be sure that all orders have been transcribed correctly.
√ Perform three valid checks on each medication.
√ Perform the Three Bedside A's (armband, allergies, assessments).
√ Document all medications after the patient has received them.

> **Assignment:** You have been assigned to administer medications to Piya Jordan, Room 403. Floor: Medical-Surgical. Period of Care 1: 0730–0815.

1. Go to the Medication Room.
2. Click on the **Automated System** (the automated dispensing device).
3. Your name and password should be entered automatically.
4. Select patient to log medications out for: Piya Jordan.

You now have access to this patient's narcotic medications.

 1. How does this reduce the potential for medication errors?

2. Select Drawer G-O on the Automated Dispensing Machine. Select *morphine sulfate*. What doses are available? Which dose is the patient currently receiving? How many mg per mL? How many mL are in the pre-filled syringe?

Pacific View Regional Hospital	MRN: 1868057	Room: 502
	Patient: Delores Gallegos	
6475 E. Duke Avenue	Sex: Female	Age: 82
	Physician: Gerald Moher, M.D.	

Physician's Orders		
Weight: 160 lbs	Age: 82	

Day/Time	Orders	Signature
Wed 1000	**Order Type:** General 1. Digoxin loading dose, to be given as follows: 0.5 mg now, then 0.25 mg every 8 hours x 2 doses; starting tomorrow, 0.125 mg PO daily. 2. Nystatin powder to rash TID. 3. Send sputum for culture and sensitivity. 4. Incentive spirometer every hour while awake. 5. Chest x-ray. 6. Add Potassium chloride 10 mEq PO daily, starting today. 7. Oncology consult.	*Gerald Moher, M.D.*

 Next you are assigned to give medications to Delores Gallegos, Room 502. Floor: Skilled Nursing. Period of Care 2: 1115–1200.

3. Look at the patient's MAR. Write down the medications she is taking and include the doses for this period of care. (Be sure to check the STAT/PREP-OP/ONE TIME section of the MAR.) Verify the MAR with the Physician's Orders. Were all of the medication orders transcribed to the MAR? What will you do if there is a discrepancy?

4. Prepare the dose of digoxin. How many tablets will you administer? How many times did you check the medication against the MAR? Did you note any discrepancies? What is your safest nursing action?

5. Go to the patient's room. Perform the Three Bedside A's before giving the digoxin. What safety check did you do before giving the digoxin?

6. *Critical Thinking:* Were you able to administer the digoxin? Why or why not? If you held the digoxin, explain your rationale. Whom will you notify if the medication is held?

The Endocrine System

HORMONES

The endocrine system is one of the body's control systems (the CNS is the other). The endocrine system produces **hormones** that regulate metabolism. These can be grouped into four basic areas:

1. Fluid balance and pH
2. Growth and development
3. Reproduction
4. Energy

Major organs of the endocrine system are:

- Hypothalamus
- Pituitary
- Thyroid
- Parathyroid
- Pancreas
- Adrenal
- Ovarian
- Testes

All of these organs secrete hormones. Hormones are chemicals that are secreted from one group of cells and exert physiologic changes on other cells. These hormones normally have an effect on distant organs. They work by negative feedback: When a hormone is needed, it is secreted. When it is not needed, it is inhibited.

97

INSULIN AND DANGERS

Insulin is a potent hormone secreted by the beta cells in the pancreas. The average adult secretes 1 to 2 units of insulin every hour. This increases to 4 to 6 units an hour after meals. When a meal is eaten, insulin secretion increases and moves glucose from the blood to muscle, liver, and fat cells. Once insulin binds to receptors on the cell's membrane, the membrane becomes permeable to glucose, and glucose rushes in. The cell can now use glucose for increased metabolism.

In a patient with diabetes mellitus, there is a chronic discrepancy between the amount of insulin required by the body and the amount available. Patients with diabetes need supplemental insulin to distribute glucose to the cells of the body and to reduce the amount of glucose in circulatory blood.

Insulin is the only effective treatment for type 1 diabetes. Insulin comes as "pork" or "human," differing by only one amino acid. Human insulin is developed in the laboratory, not from human pancreatic cells. It is called *human* insulin because it is identical to that developed in the human body. U-100 insulin is the main concentration used in the United States. It is 100 units of insulin per mL. When U-100 insulin is administered, it must be measured with a U-100 insulin syringe.

Insulin must be within the expiration date to be effective. Many errors in insulin administration are made because the insulin is out of date. ***Always check the expiration date on the insulin vial before drawing up a dose.***

HIGH-ALERT MEDICATIONS

Insulin is one of the medications most often involved in medication errors. The group of medications most often involved in errors is referred to as high-alert medications. These medications need special care when ordering, dispensing, stocking, and administering. These medications include:

- Insulin
- Potassium chloride
- Fentanyl
- Lasix
- Heparin
- Morphine

For a nurse administering high-alert medications, it is good practice to always have a second RN check that you are administering the *correct amount* of the *correct medication*. The nurse administering the medication draws up the dose and then validates with the second nurse both the vial and the syringe to verify that the medication and the amount are correct.

Case Scenarios

A student nurse was administering medications and needed to administer 10 units of regular insulin. When she drew it up in the insulin syringe, it just didn't "look like enough," so she drew up 100 units instead. She administered all 100 units to her patient, who had a severe insulin reaction and needed runs of dextrose to counteract the overdose of insulin.

One of the most dangerous high-alert medications is *potassium chloride*. Many patients need potassium replacement, often because of diuretics which deplete potassium levels. Potassium can be given po (by mouth) but is often ordered IV for faster results. It can be infused IV in a primary IV bag. For example, the prescriber may order *1000 mL D_5W with 20 mEq KCl at 100 mL/hr*. Or if the patient's potassium level is very low, the doctor may order "runs" of potassium, that is, *10 mEq of KCl in 100 mL D_5W over 1 hour*. Because potassium chloride is ordered so routinely on many units, the drug was part of the unit's "stock" of medications. The problem comes when a doctor or nurse infuses too much potassium chloride too quickly or grabs a potassium chloride vial, mistaking it for normal saline, and uses it to flush a patient's IV line. Potassium, when infused too rapidly, can cause severe adverse cardiac effects and often death.

Because of manufacturing, potassium chloride vials look very similar to *normal saline* vials. This, in itself, accounts for a multitude of errors. Because of the vast amount of errors related to potassium chloride administration, the hospital's accrediting body, Joint Commission on Accreditation of Healthcare Organizations (JCAHO), has recommended the removal of concentrated potassium chloride from "stock" medications.

Another problem with potassium chloride is confusion with Lasix. When a patient is receiving Lasix (a diuretic), the potassium level may fall. A patient who is receiving Lasix is often taking potassium chloride replacements. Most nurses study these drugs together in their pharmacology courses and, as a result, they may confuse the two drugs (a "cognitive mix-up"). This results in a nurse substituting one medication for another.

Case Scenarios

An elderly man was transferred from a long-term care facility with pneumonia and CHF. The physician ordered 40 mg of Lasix IVP. As the nurse completed the injection, she realized she had administered 40 mEq of potassium chloride. The patient had a cardiac arrest and died.

Pacific View Regional Hospital **6475 E. Duke Avenue**	**MRN:** 1868065 **Patient:** Stacey Crider	**Room:** 202
	Sex: Female	**Age:** 21
	Physician: John Shelby, M.D.	

Physician's Orders

Weight: 214 lbs   **Age:** 21

Day/Time	Orders	Signature
Tue 1900	**Order Type:** General	*Albert Song, M.D.*
	1. Change Insulin Lispro to use premeal algorithm: Breakfast: If premeal glucose is:	
	2. <60: Give 18 Units 61-80: Give 19 Units 81-100: Give 20 Units	
	3. 101-130: Give 22 Units 131-160: Give 24 Units 161-200: Give 26 Units >200 call MD	
	4. Lunch: If premeal glucose is: <60: Give 14 Units 61-80: Give 15 Units	
	5. 81-100: Give 16 Units 101-130: Give 18 Units 131-160: Give 20 Units	
	6. 161-200: Give 22 Units >200 call MD	
	7. Dinner: If premeal glucose is: <60: Give 10 Units 61-80: Give 11 Units	
	8. 81-100: Give 12 Units 101-130: Give 14 Units 131-160: Give 16 Units	

	MRN: 1868065	Room: 202
Pacific View Regional Hospital	Patient: Stacey Crider	
6475 E. Duke Avenue	Sex: Female	Age: 21
	Physician: John Shelby, M.D.	

Physician's Orders

Weight: 214 lbs   **Age:** 21

Day/Time	Orders	Signature
Tue 0630	**Order Type:** General	*John Shelby, M.D.*
	1. Admit to Perinatal services.	
	2. Diagnosis: Intrauterine pregnancy of 27.4 weeks, Obesity, Gestational Diabetes with poor control, Preterm labor, and Bacterial Vaginosis.	
	3. Diet: Carbohydrate controlled as recommended by Nutrition consult.	
	4. Activity: Bedrest, strict I & O.	
	5. Fluids: Restrict total to 2400 mL/day while on Magnesium sulfate therapy.	
	6. IV of Lactated Ringer's at 30 mL/hr. 0.45% NS (500 mL) with Magnesium sulfate (50 g) at rate to control uterine activity (2 g/hr = 20 mL/hr).	
	7. Begin Magnesium sulfate IV now. Give 4 g bolus over 30 min then give 2 g/hr.	
	8. Continuous EFM and document FHR and contractions every hour.	
	9. Notify MD for abnormal fetal heart rate or uterine contractions greater than 5 in 1 hour.	
	10. Double patient's usual dose of insulin for the next 72 hours.	
		cont. next page

Pacific View Regional Hospital 6475 E. Duke Avenue	MRN: 1868065 Room: 202 Patient: Stacey Crider Sex: Female Age: 21 Physician: John Shelby, M.D.

Physician's Orders (cont.)

Weight: 214 lbs   **Age:** 21

Day/Time	Orders	Signature
Tue 0630	**Order Type:** General 11. Doubled doses are: NPH 42 Units subQ at bedtime. Lispro 20 Units subQ prebreakfast. Lispro 16 Units subQ prelunch. Lispro 12 Units subQ predinner. 12. Metronidazole 500 mg PO BID for 7 days. 13. Prenatal multivitamin 1 PO daily. 14. Give Betamethasone 12 mg IM every 24 hours for total of 2 doses. 15. Bedside testing of fasting capillary blood glucose (before meals)and 1 hour after beginning meal wtih targets of: Premeal <95, 1 hour postmeal <135.	*John Shelby, M.D.*

EXERCISE 1

 You will be going to Pacific View Regional Hospital to administer medications for your assigned patient. Please remember when administering medications to all patients:

√ Check the MAR against the physician's order to be sure that all orders have been transcribed correctly.
√ Perform three valid checks on each medication.
√ Perform the Three Bedside A's (armband, allergies, assessments).
√ Document all medications after the patient has received them.

> **Assignment:** You have been assigned to administer medications to Stacey Crider, Room 202. Floor: Obstetrics. Period of Care 1: 0730–0815.

 1. Write down the types of insulin this patient receives.

2. Look up *insulin* in the Drug Guide. List the peak times for both types of insulin.

3. Prepare the medications for this period of care. Prepare the insulin injection. What type of insulin and syringe will you use? What is important to note about each?

4. Insulin is a high-alert medication. What does this mean? As the nurse administering this medication, you should perform what special safety check?

The Reproductive System

FEMALE REPRODUCTION

Oral contraceptives are widely used because of the ease of use and their effectiveness to prevent pregnancy. There are two major types of oral contraceptives:

1. The "pill," which is an estrogen-progestin combination
2. The "mini-pill," which is progestin only

The combination pill is the most effective in preventing pregnancy. These drugs inhibit ovulation and make the endometrial environment hostile to sperm.

It is very important to teach women that the effectiveness of oral contraception is easily compromised by the use of other drugs, including over-the-counter (OTC) medications. Some examples of drugs that may inhibit the "pill's" effectiveness include:

- Tylenol (acetaminophen)
- Antibiotics
- Antihistamines/decongestants
- Caffeine
- Antidepressants

(Kee JL, Hayes ER: *Pharmacology: a nursing process approach*, ed 4, Philadelphia, 2003, W.B. Saunders.)

When oral contraceptives were first introduced in the 1960s, there were many difficult adverse effects, especially circulatory disorders. Since then, the effectiveness of lower dosaging has made the use of oral contraceptives as safe as pregnancy.

Pacific View Regional Hospital **6475 E. Duke Avenue**	**MRN:** 1868048	**Room:** 402
	Patient: Jacquline Catanazaro	
	Sex: Female	**Age:** 45
	Physician: Howard Steele, M.D.	

Physician's Orders

Weight: 186 lbs **Age:** 45

Day/Time	Orders	Signature
Mon 1600	**Order Type:** General	*Howard Steele, M.D.*
	1. Admit to Medical Unit.	
	2. Regular diet.	
	3. Encourage fluids.	
	4. Vital signs including oxygen saturation every 2 hours for first 4 hours, then every 4 hours.	
	5. PEFR every 4 hours.	
	6. Activity up as tolerated; encourage ambulation.	
	7. O2 at 2L/min via nasal cannula.	
	8. Beclomethasone (84 mcg/puff) via MDI, 2 puffs every 6 hours.	
	9. Albuterol 5 mg via nebulizer every 6 hours.	
	10. Ipratropium bromide (18 mcg/puff) via MDI, 2 puffs every 6 hours to be administered following Albuterol.	
	11. Amoxicillin 500 mg IV in 100 mL D5W every 6 hours today.	
	12. Psychiatric consult.	
	13. IV of D5W at 125 mL/hr.	

Pacific View Regional Hospital	MRN: 1868048 Room: 402
	Patient: Jacquline Catanazaro
6475 E. Duke Avenue	Sex: Female Age: 45
	Physician: Howard Steele, M.D.

Physician's Orders

Weight:	Age:

Day/Time	Orders	Signature
Mon 1005	**Order Type:** Emergency Room Orders 1. Oxygen at 2L/min with continuous pulse oximetry. 2. IV of D5W at 125 mL/hr. 3. Methylprednisolone sodium succinate 120 mg in 150 mL D5W x 1 now. 4. Albuterol 5 mg and Ipratropium bromide 0.5 mg by nebulizer x 1 now. If wheezing remains, repeat dose x 1. 5. Labs STAT: ABG, CBC, Sputum culture, and U/A. 6. Chest x-ray STAT.	*Arthur Kelley, M.D*

EXERCISE 1

 You will be going to Pacific View Regional Hospital to administer medications for your assigned patient. Please remember when administering medications to all patients:

√ Check the MAR against the physician's order to be sure that all orders have been transcribed correctly.
√ Perform three valid checks on each medication.
√ Perform the Three Bedside A's (armband, allergies, assessments).
√ Document all medications after the patient has received them.

Assignment: You have been assigned to administer medications to Jacquline Catanzaro, Room 402. Floor: Medical-Surgical. Period of Care 1: 0730–0815.

 1. List medications the patient is currently receiving.

2. Look up the listed medications in the Drug Guide provided, noting the classification, safe dose range, and nursing implications.

3. What antibiotic is the patient currently taking? What is the dose?

4. If the patient were being discharged home and takes birth control pills, what do you need to teach her?

PREGNANCY

When a pregnant woman ingests a drug, it is transported across the placenta into fetal circulation. Fetal blood levels reach 50–100% of the amount of the drug in the mother's circulation. The drug is then excreted into the amniotic fluid and, in swallowing some of the amniotic fluid, the fetus is reexposed to the drug. The blood-brain barrier in the fetus is not fully developed, and much of the drug molecules may enter the fetal brain and cause anatomical malformations.

It is important that you educate your patients on the dangers of the following drugs during pregnancy:

1. Alcohol—can cause fetal alcohol syndrome (FAS), with multiple congenital defects and mental retardation
2. Cigarette smoke—can cause fetal hypoxia and mental retardation
3. Marijuana—impairs DNA and RNA and oxygen levels
4. Caffeine—can cause spontaneous abortions, preterm labor, and "small-for-gestational-age" infants

MALE REPRODUCTION

Sexual dysfunction may include inhibited sexual desire, erectile dysfunction, ejaculatory dysfunction, or failure of detumescence. Many drugs may cause erectile dysfunction, including:

- Some antihypertensives
- Some antidepressants
- Cimetidine (antiulcer)
- Some chemotherapy drugs
- Alcohol/marijuana

Drugs Used to *Treat* Sexual Dysfunction:

1. l-dopa (Parkinson's drug) may stimulate libido and erectile function.
2. MAO inhibitors may aid in treatment of premature ejaculation.
3. Antiimpotence agents (Viagra) help restore erectile response.

TOO FAMILIAR VERSUS TOO FOREIGN

A certain degree of anxiety keeps us on our toes. Being comfortable and confident in our patient care area can actually be detrimental to patient safety, and administering multiple "routine" medications may actually lead to medication errors. When the nurse knows the patients and their medications, it is easy to be negligent. The nurse may be embarrassed to check the patient's ID band again, wanting the patient to have confidence and comfort in the nurse.

With the increasing numbers of new medications, the nurse may be totally unfamiliar with a drug, making that drug "foreign" to the nurse.

Being too comfortable can be a problem, if the nurse becomes negligent. Being too familiar can cause a problem, and so can the concept of too *foreign*.

INCREASING NUMBER OF NEW DRUGS

With Viagra and other new medications being introduced to the market and available in the patient care area at a rapid rate, nurses need to be familiar with more and more drug information. There are approximately 8,000 drug products available today, as compared with 656 products that were in use in 1961.

(Pepper GA: Errors in drug administration by nurses, *Am J Health-System Pharm* 52:390-5, 1995.)

There are too many drugs for nurses to recognize, understand, and safely administer based on memory. Hospital units need up-to-date drug references, and nurses need to use them. If you don't know what you are giving, that the dose is safe, and what you need to do to keep your patient safe, this is another potential for a medication error. In addition to drug references, units need Internet access so that a nurse can research any medication not yet in the drug reference books.

With the increasing number of generic drugs, the unique appearance of a drug that the nurse may have recognized may now be entirely different. You can no longer depend on the pill's appearance. A small white, round pill the pharmacist always identified as metoprolol (Lopressor) may now be a large pink pill.

> *As long as a medication is protected under patent, it's fairly easy to identify it by shape and color, but once it becomes generic and is made by multiple manufacturers, it can be sold in a variety of colors and shapes. The system is generating confusion.*
>
> *(Lewis P: Nursing, medical errors and the health care system: What's gone wrong? Can it be fixed?, Texas Medical Center News, Vol 22, December 1, 2000.)*

The nurse who always knew that Lopressor was a small white pill has had to adapt to the fact that the institution is now ordering from a cheaper manufacturer, and Lopressor looks different.

Pacific View Regional Hospital 6475 E. Duke Avenue	MRN: 1868057	Room: 502
	Patient: Delores Gallegos	
	Sex: Female	Age: 82
	Physician: Gerald Moher, M.D.	

Physician's Orders

Weight: 160 lbs   **Age:** 82

Day/Time	Orders	Signature
Mon 1400	**Order Type:** General	*Gerald Moher, M.D.*

Order Type: General

1. Admit to Skilled Nursing Unit, Internal Medicine Service.

2. Activity: Up ad lib.

3. Diet: Regular, low salt pending Dietary consult recommendations.

4. Dietary consult.

5. Skin care TID to rash.

6. Intake and Output every 8 hours.

7. Vital signs every 8 hours.

8. Labs: Basic metabolic panel every other day to include sodium, potassium, chloride, CO2, blood urea nitrogen, glucose, creatinine.

9. Furosemide 40 mg PO daily.

10. Captopril 12.5 mg PO TID.

11. Metoprolol 25 mg PO daily.

12. Docusate sodium 100 mg PO daily.

13. Bisacodyl 10 mg daily prn no bowel movement per rectum.

14. Daily weight.

Pacific View Regional Hospital 6475 E. Duke Avenue	MRN: 1868057	Room: 502
	Patient: Delores Gallegos	
	Sex: Female	Age: 82
	Physician: Gerald Moher, M.D.	

Physician's Orders		

Weight:	Age:	

Day/Time	Orders	Signature
Wed 0730	**Order Type:** General 1. Acetaminophen 650 mg PO/PR every 4 hours prn T > 101.3 F. (telephone order)	*Gerald Moher, M.D.*

EXERCISE 2

 You will be going to Pacific View Regional Hospital to administer medications for your assigned patient. Please remember when administering medications to all patients:

√ Check the MAR against the physician's order to be sure that all orders have been transcribed correctly.
√ Perform three valid checks on each medication.
√ Perform the Three Bedside A's (armband, allergies, assessments).
√ Document all medications after the patient has received them.

Assignment: You have been assigned to administer medications to Delores Gallegos, Room 502. Floor: Skilled Nursing. Period of Care 1: 0730–0815.

 1. Write down all of the medications the patient is receiving.

2. When you compared the medications ordered by the doctor with the MAR, did you note any discrepancies?

3. How many milligrams of captopril are ordered? What doses are available? How many tablets will you administer of which dose?

4. *Critical Thinking:* Related to question 3, what is your safest nursing action?

GI/Nutrition

The digestive system consists of the alimentary canal and the digestive tract, beginning at the oral cavity and ending at the anus. The organs of the digestive system include:

- Oral cavity
- Esophagus
- Stomach
- Small intestine
- Large intestine
- Pancreas
- Gall bladder
- Liver

DISTURBANCES IN THE GI SYSTEM

Peptic Ulcer

This is a term used for an ulceration in the esophagus, stomach, or duodenum. The ulcer is named for the area of involvement.

Gastroesophageal Reflux Disease (GERD)

Esophagitis or esophageal ulceration caused by regurgitation of gastric content into the esophagus.

Drugs Used to Treat Acid/Peptic Disorders

1. Antacids—Neutralize hydrochloric acid and reduce pepsin production (Maalox, Mylanta).
2. Helicobacter (*H. pylori*) agents—Antimicrobials, like amoxicillin or tetracycline, or combination antimicrobial and antisecretory agent.
3. Histamine H_2-receptor antagonists—Compete with histamine for binding sites on the parietal cells. Without histamine binding and stimulating these cells, hydrochloric acid production is blocked (cimetidine, ranitidine).
4. Proton pump inhibitors—Antisecretory substances, which block the final step of acid production; e.g., lansoprazole (Prevacid), omeprazole (Prilosec), esomeprazole (Nexium).

Case Scenarios

A physician ordered Maalox 30 mL to be inserted 3 times a day into a patient's peg (feeding) tube. When the nurse attempted to inject the medication with a large-bore "Toomey" syringe, the ends did not fit together. So the nurse chose another syringe with a smaller-bore needle end and infused the 30 mL of Maalox. What the nurse did not realize was that she inserted the Maalox into the patient's central venous line in error. The patient died.

Pacific View Regional Hospital **6475 E. Duke Avenue**	**MRN:** 1868011 **Patient:** Clarence Hughes **Sex:** Male **Physician:** Thomas Price, M.D.	**Room:** 404 **Age:** 73

Physician's Orders

Weight: 207 lbs   **Age:** 73

Day/Time	Orders	Signature
Tue 0600	**Order Type:** General	*Thomas Price, M.D.*
	1. Discontinue Foley catheter this morning, may straight cath every 6-8 hours if unable to void.	
	2. Discontinue cryocuff.	
	3. Change dressing every day and prn.	
	4. Activity: Up to chair twice a day. Physical therapy to ambulate.	
	5. Discontinue IV infusion; convert to a saline lock.	
	6. Discontinue Morphine PCA.	
	7. Discontinue Cefazolin after 6th dose.	
	8. Oxycodone with acetaminophen 1-2 tablets PO every 4-6 hours prn for pain.	
	9. Labs: Hemoglobin, hematocrit and prothrombin tomorrow morning.	

Pacific View Regional Hospital	MRN: 1868011	Room: 404
	Patient: Clarence Hughes	
6475 E. Duke Avenue	Sex: Male	Age: 73
	Physician: Thomas Price, M.D.	

Physician's Orders

Weight: 207 lbs   **Age:** 73

Day/Time	Orders	Signature
Mon 0715	**Order Type:** General	*Myron Kuhn, M.D.*
	1. Monitor vital signs and circulation, motion, and sensation every 8 hours.	
	2. Wean off oxygen with oxygen saturation greater than 90% on room air.	
	3. Continuous passive motion (CPM) machine 6 hours per day to L knee with the following goals: 45 degrees postop day 1 60 degrees postop day 2 75 degrees postop day 3 90 degrees postop day 4 Notify MD if unable to meet goals as specified.	
	4. Patient to be out of CPM at night; L leg should be flat with pillow under the heel.	
	5. Activity: Up in chair today before noon. Physical therapy to ambulate this afternoon.	
	6. Decrease IV infusion to 30 mL/hr if patient is taking adequate oral fluids.	
	7. Enoxaparin 30 mg subQ every 12 hours to start this evening.	
	8. Labs: Hemoglobin, hematocrit, and prothrombin tomorrow morning.	

Pacific View Regional Hospital	MRN: 1868011	Room: 404
	Patient: Clarence Hughes	
6475 E. Duke Avenue	Sex: Male	Age: 73
	Physician: Thomas Price, M.D.	

Physician's Orders

Weight: 207 lbs		Age: 73

Day/Time	Orders	Signature
Sun 1600	**Order Type:** Postoperative 1. Admit to the Medical Surgical floor--diagnosis status post left total knee arthroplasty. 2. Diet: Clear liquids tonight; advance to regular diet as tolerated. 3. Vital signs every 4 hours including circulation, motion and sensation checks. 4. Intake and Output measurement every 8 hours. 5. Oxygen 2L flow by nasal cannula. 6. Incentive spirometer 10 times every hour while awake. 7. Activity: Bedrest. 8. Foley catheter to gravity drainage. 9. Wound drain--hemovac to compression suction. 10. Reinforce dressing to L knee as needed. 11. Cryocuff to left knee. Sequential compression device to R leg while in bed. 12. IV D5.45 NS with 20 mEq KCl per liter to infuse at 125 mL/hr. 13. Cefazolin 2 grams IV every 8 hours X 6 doses. 14. Morphine sulfate IV PCA 1 mg every 10 minutes/lock out 24 mg every 4 hours.	*Thomas Price, M.D.* cont. next page

Pacific View Regional Hospital	MRN: 1868011	Room: 404
	Patient: Clarence Hughes	
6475 E. Duke Avenue	Sex: Male	Age: 73
	Physician: Thomas Price, M.D.	

Physician's Orders *(cont.)*

Weight: 207 lbs   **Age:** 73

Day/Time	Orders	Signature
Sun 1600	**Order Type:** Postoperative	*Thomas Price, M.D.*
	15. Docusate sodium 100 mg PO BID.	
	16. Celecoxib 100 mg PO BID.	
	17. Timolol maleate 0.25% ophthalmic solution 2 drops to both eyes every 12 hours.	
	18. Pilocarpine 1% ophthalmic solution 2 drops to both eyes every 12 hours.	
	19. Promethazine 12.5 to 25 mg IV every 6 hours prn for nausea.	
	20. Aluminum hydroxide with magnesium and simethicone 30 mL PO every 8 hours prn for gastrointestinal upset.	
	21. Bisacodyl 10 mg suppository per rectum every 12 hours prn for constipation.	
	22. Milk of magnesia 30 mL PO every 8 hours prn for constipation.	
	23. Acetaminophen 325-650 mg PO every 4-6 hours prn for fever >101 F.	
	24. Temazepam 15 mg PO at bedtime prn for sleep.	
	25. Labs: Hemoglobin and hematocrit in morning.	

EXERCISE 1

 You will be going to Pacific View Regional Hospital to administer medications to your assigned patient. Please remember when administering medications to all patients:

√ Check the MAR against the physician's order to be sure that all orders have been transcribed correctly.
√ Perform three valid checks on each medication.
√ Perform the Three Bedside A's (armband, allergies, assessments).
√ Document all medications after the patient has received them.

Assignment: You have been assigned to administer medications to Clarence Hughes, Room 404. Floor: Medical-Surgical. Period of Care 1: 0730–0815.

 1. List all the medications the patient is currently receiving.

2. What medications is the patient receiving for constipation? How is the po liquid drug ordered? What information do you know from the label? According to the *amount* of solution, what is the *dose* you are giving?

Pacific View Regional Hospital	MRN: 1868018	Room: 302
	Patient: Tommy Douglas	
6475 E. Duke Avenue	Sex: Male	Age: 6
	Physician: Robert Gardner, M.D.	

Physician's Orders

Weight:	Age: 6	

Day/Time	Orders	Signature
Sun 2300	**Order Type:** Transfer	*Robert Gardner, M.D.*

Order Type: Transfer

1. Admit to the Intensive Care Unit.
   Diagnosis: Traumatic Brain Injury, status post ventriculostomy placement, condition critical.

2. Vital signs q1h, head of bed up 30 degrees, keep head midline, cervical collar, ICP precautions.

3. Neurosurgery/neurology consults.

4. Neuro vital signs every 30 minutes. Hourly when stable. ICP monitoring.

5. Radial arterial line to infuse Normal saline with Heparin 1 unit/mL at 3 mL/hr for ABG draws.

6. Saline lock with flushes 3-5 mL IV every 4-6 hours as needed to keep patent.

7. Cefazolin 500 mg IV every 6 hours (100 mg/kg/day).

8. IV of Normal saline at 40 mL/hr.

9. Mannitol 20 g IV every 6 hours.

10. Ranitidine 20 mg IV every 6 hours.

11. Labs: ABGs, electrolytes, type and cross match for 2 units PRBCs STAT.
    Chest x-ray now and every morning.

12. Ventilator settings:
    SIMV/Vc, FiO_2 = 0.40, IMV = 18, VT = 200, Ti = 0.7, PEEP 0, PS = 5. Use end tidal CO_2 monitor.

➡ Next proceed to Tommy Douglas, Room 302. Floor: Pediatrics. Period of Care 2: 1115–1200.

3. *Critical Thinking:* This patient has ranitidine 20 mg IV available. What is the drug classification? How does this drug work to reduce gastric reflux? Verify this medication on the Physician's transfer orders. Is this a safe dose? What is the safest nursing action?

8

Chemotherapy

ANTINEOPLASTIC DRUGS

Antineoplastic drugs, introduced into the treatment of cancer in the 1940s, cause cell death by interfering with cancer cell replication. They may be given for cure, control, or palliation. They may be used alone or in conjunction with radiation or surgery. There are several types of antineoplastic drugs in use:

1. Alkylating agents
2. Antimetabolites
3. Antitumor antibiotics
4. Plant alkaloids
5. Cytoprotectants
6. Miscellaneous antineoplastic agents

Patients receiving antineoplastics must be closely monitored for side effects. In the process of destroying malignant cells, chemotherapy suppresses bone marrow, resulting in low WBC and platelet counts. It causes anorexia, nausea and vomiting, diarrhea, stomatitis, alopecia, and infertility.

As a nurse administering chemotherapeutic agents,* you will need to monitor your patient's blood work closely. Patients with bone marrow suppression are very suscepti-ble to infection and may be placed on protective (reverse) isolation. This protects the patient from invading microorganisms from staff, visitors, and other patients in the health care setting.

*Anytime an intravenous chemotherapy drug is administered, the medication and dose should be checked with another nurse.

125

LOOK-ALIKE AND SOUND-ALIKE MEDICATIONS

One factor that can contribute to errors in medication administration is the problem of *look-alike* and *sound-alike* drugs. Errors related to this problem can occur at any point of the "drug therapy chain." The prescriber may order the incorrect drug. The pharmacist may dispense the incorrect drug. The nurse may administer the incorrect drug. You may think this type of error is easily avoidable (especially if the nurse is following the "three valid checks" and the "Three Bedside A's"). However, with "confirmation bias," as previously described, the person hearing the order may complete the order with what they *thought* they heard.

Case Scenarios

A physician ordered Parizac, which was not listed in the formulary (the book that lists all of the medications a hospital carries). The pharmacist transcribed the order as Prozac, which was familiar to him. Both drugs came in the same strength (20-mg capsules), which exacerbated the error.

There are many drugs whose names are very similar and whose doses are identical. This is the cause for a number of errors and potential errors in medication administration. There are more than 600 pairs of look-alike or sound-alike medications. Examples of medication names that have caused confusion:

Zantac		Zyrtec
Flomax		Volmax
Colazal		Clorazil
Celebrex	Cerebyx	Celexa
Narcan		Norcuron
Noroxin		Neurontin
Heparin		Hespan

Some Name **and** Dosing Confusion:

Quinine 200 mg	Quinidine 200 mg
Sulfasalazine 500 mg	Sulfadiazine 500 mg
Hydroxyzine 25 mg	Hydralazine 25 mg
Losec 20 mg	Lasix 20 mg

Check *http://www.usp.org* for a complete list of problem names from the United States Pharmacopia (USP).

Case Scenarios

A doctor ordered Hespan (a plasma expander) for a patient in CCU being treated for bleeding. The nurse mistakenly selected a bag of heparin (an anticoagulant) 25,000 units in 500 cc. The patient received the entire bag at 11:00 a.m. and another at 2:00 p.m. The patient hemorrhaged and died.

Chemotherapeutic drugs are among those drugs that are most toxic and often involved in medication errors.

Case Scenarios

A physician ordered a 64-year-old woman to receive carboplatin (Paraplatin), a chemotherapy drug. Because of a pharmacy mix-up, she received cisplatin (Platinol) in error. She died as a result of the mix-up.

Case Scenarios

In one hospital, five patients experienced respiratory arrest within a 7 1/2-hour period. It was later discovered that a pharmacy technician had actually put an antibiotic label on a potent paralyzing drug and covered the manufacturer's warning label with the pharmacy label.

As you can see, many medication errors occur not only with chemotherapeutic drugs but also as a result of any break in the drug therapy chain. The last two errors resulted from pharmacy errors, but it was the nurse who was ultimately responsible for administering the wrong drug.

Pacific View Regional Hospital	MRN: 1868051	Room: 503
	Patient: Kathryn Doyle	
6475 E. Duke Avenue	Sex: Female	Age: 79
	Physician: Gerald Moher, M.D.	

Physician's Orders

Weight: 105 lbs   **Age:** 79

Day/Time	Orders	Signature
Mon 1000	**Order Type:** Transfer 1. Admit to Skilled Nursing Unit, Internal Medicine. 2. Diet: Regular, soft mechanical. 3. Vital signs every 8 hours. 4. Activity: Ambulate at least four times a day. Patient needs to get up to use bathroom. 5. Physical therapy to direct rehabilitation. 6. Dietary consult. 7. Social work consult. 8. Calcium citrate 2 tablets PO BID. 9. Ferrous sulfate 325 mg PO TID with meals. 10. Docusate sodium 100 mg PO daily. 11. Ibuprofen 600 mg PO TID. 12. Oxycodone 2.5 mg with acetaminophen 325 mg 1 or 2 tablets PO every 4-6 hours prn for pain. 13. Acetaminophen 325-650 mg PO every 4 hours prn for mild pain or fever >101.5 F. 14. Daily weight.	*Gerald Moher, M.D.*

EXERCISE 1

 You will be going to Pacific View Regional Hospital to administer medications for your assigned patient. Please remember when administering medications to all patients:

√ Check the MAR against the physician's order to be sure that all orders have been transcribed correctly.
√ Perform three valid checks on each medication.
√ Perform the Three Bedside A's (armband, allergies, assessments).
√ Document all medications after the patient has received them.

Assignment: You have been assigned to administer medications to Kathryn Doyle, Room 503. Floor: Skilled Nursing. Period of Care 1: 0730–0815.

 1. List all medications ordered for this patient from the MAR. Review the list with the original physician's order. Are all medication orders clear and complete? Is any needed information missing?

2. Prepare the patient's calcium citrate. Compare the physician's order for this medication with the MAR. Compare the MAR with what's available in the patient's drawer. Describe any inconsistency.

3. If the order is not complete, but the drug is available in the patient's drawer, what is the safest nursing action? Can the pharmacist verify this order for you?

4. Check *acetaminophen*. How many different doses are in the drawer?

5. *Critical Thinking:* What assessments will you make to determine whether the patient should receive acetaminophen? How will you determine which dose to give? If the maximum dose of acetaminophen is 4 grams in 24 hours, how many doses can the patient receive?

Antiinfectives

Microorganisms attach to host cell receptor sites and invade the tissue, multiply, and produce an infection. Microorganisms that produce disease are called *pathogenic*. These pathogenic microorganisms can be:

1. Bacteria
2. Viruses
3. Fungi

Bacteria are classified as:

- Aerobic (requiring oxygen)
- Anaerobic (cannot live with oxygen)
- Gram-positive (will "take" gram stain)
- Gram-negative (will not "take" gram stain)
- Shape (cocci versus bacilli)

Viruses are parasites living inside the cell.

Fungi are plantlike organisms that live as either a *parasite* (feeding on a living organism) or *saprophyte* (living on decaying organic matter).

INFECTION

An infectious disease occurs when a pathogen is present and causes clinical symptoms of an infection. Diagnosing an infection involves identification of the organism by:

- *Culture*—Growing the microorganism in the lab and identifying its appearance, shape, gram stain, and color.
- *Serology*—Measures the antibody level (titer) to a specific organism.

131

ANTIBIOTIC-RESISTANT MICROORGANISMS

Increasing numbers of microorganisms are resistant to antibiotic therapy. Bacteria are developing mutant strains that are "resistant" to particular antibiotics. It is thought that these resistant bacteria have developed thickened cell walls, possibly by overuse of broad-spectrum antibiotics.

ANTIINFECTIVE DRUGS

Antibacterial (antibiotic) drugs are used to stop bacterial infections. They work to either kill the microorganism (bactericidal) or inhibit its growth (bacteriostatic).

Antibiotics are:

1. Broad-spectrum—Effective against several groups of microorganisms.
2. Narrow-spectrum—Effective against a limited group of microorganisms.

Identification of the causative microorganism for an infection usually takes time. A patient is often started on *empiric* therapy. This is therapy in which the antibiotic most often used to treat this type of infection is started immediately. Before *any antibiotic* is started, however, the patient should have a *culture and sensitivity* obtained. Once an organism is identified, it is tested in the lab with various antibiotics to see which will be most effective. Then *directed* therapy is started, using the antibiotic identified as the most effective, the antibiotic to which the organism is *susceptible*.

SAFETY ISSUES INVOLVED WITH ANTIBIOTICS

Many patients are allergic to penicillin, and the allergy can be a deadly one. If administering penicillin to a patient, be sure to determine that the patient is NOT allergic to penicillin. (Remember the second Bedside A.) There is also the issue of "cross-sensitivity." This occurs when a patient who is allergic to a medication receives a drug that has some properties of the medication to which he or she is allergic. This occurs with a group of drugs known as cephalosporins, which are structurally and pharmacologically related to penicillin. Patients with severe allergies to penicillin may also be allergic to cephalosporins.

Another group of antibiotics with special safety issues is aminoglycosides. They were originally used in the treatment of tuberculosis and are a very potent group of antibiotics. They can kill both gram-positive and gram-negative bacteria. Aminoglycosides are not absorbed from the GI tract and so are given IV. They should not be given if a less toxic drug would be effective. This group of drugs is both *ototoxic* and *nephrotoxic*.

Case Scenarios

A patient with a fungal infection (cutaneous candidiasis) of the buttocks was ordered to have nystatin ointment (antifungal) to his buttocks tid. The nurse applied nitroglycerin ointment (vasodilator) instead. The patient died.

This error occurred because of a "system" failure. The staff routinely left the nystatin ointment at the bedside to apply after bathing. The nitroglycerin ointment was left there as well, and the nurse did not perform three valid checks on the medication.

Pacific View Regional Hospital 6475 E. Duke Avenue	MRN: 1868018 Room: 302 Patient: Tommy Douglas Sex: Male Age: 6 Physician: Robert Gardner, M.D.

Physician's Orders

Weight:	Age: 6	
Day/Time	**Orders**	**Signature**
Wed 0730	**Order Type:** General 1. Normal saline 400 ml IV bolus STAT. 2. Sodium bicarbonate 20 mEq IV STAT. 3. Repeat ABG in 30 minutes. 4. Restart Vasopressin IV at 10 units/hr. 5. Increase Norepinephrine IV to 0.15 mcg/kg/min.	*Gene Sandoval, M.D.*

Pacific View Regional Hospital	MRN: 1868018	Room: 302
	Patient: Tommy Douglas	
6475 E. Duke Avenue	Sex: Male	Age: 6
	Physician: Robert Gardner, M.D.	

Physician's Orders

Weight: **Age:** 6

Day/Time	Orders	Signature
Mon 2100	**Order Type:** General 1. Acetaminophen 200 mg via nasogastric tube every 4 hours prn temperature >101.5 F. 2. Artificial tears with drops as needed to both eyes every 4 hours.	*Robert Gardner, M.D.*

Pacific View Regional Hospital	MRN: 1868018	Room: 302
	Patient: Tommy Douglas	
6475 E. Duke Avenue	Sex: Male	Age: 6
	Physician: Robert Gardner, M.D.	

Physician's Orders

Weight: **Age:** 6

Day/Time	Orders	Signature
Mon 0700	**Order Type:** General 1. Normal saline 200 mL IV bolus x 1 now. 2. Lidocaine 2% solution 0.5 mL instilled into endotracheal tube prior to suctioning. 3. Increase IMV to 25.	*Robert Gardner, M.D.*

Pacific View Regional Hospital	MRN: 1868018	Room: 302
	Patient: Tommy Douglas	
6475 E. Duke Avenue	Sex: Male	Age: 6
	Physician: Robert Gardner, M.D.	

Physician's Orders

Weight:	Age: 6	

Day/Time	Orders	Signature
Sun 2300	**Order Type:** Transfer	Robert Gardner, M.D.

1. Admit to the Intensive Care Unit.
   Diagnosis: Traumatic Brain Injury, status post ventriculostomy placement, condition critical.

2. Vital signs q1h, head of bed up 30 degrees, keep head midline, cervical collar, ICP precautions.

3. Neurosurgery/neurology consults.

4. Neuro vital signs every 30 minutes. Hourly when stable. ICP monitoring.

5. Radial arterial line to infuse Normal saline with Heparin 1 unit/mL at 3 mL/hr for ABG draws.

6. Saline lock with flushes 3-5 mL IV every 4-6 hours as needed to keep patent.

7. Cefazolin 500 mg IV every 6 hours (100 mg/kg/day).

8. IV of Normal saline at 40 mL/hr.

9. Mannitol 20 g IV every 6 hours.

10. Ranitidine 20 mg IV every 6 hours.

11. Labs: ABGs, electrolytes, type and cross match for 2 units PRBCs STAT.
    Chest x-ray now and every morning.

12. Ventilator settings:
    SIMV/Vc, FiO2 = 0.40, IMV = 18, VT = 200, Ti = 0.7, PEEP 0, PS = 5. Use end tidal CO_2 monitor.

EXERCISE 1

 You will be going to Pacific View Regional Hospital to administer medications for your assigned patient. Please remember when administering medications to all patients:

√   Check the MAR against the physician's order to be sure that all orders have been transcribed correctly.
√   Perform three valid checks on each medication.
√   Perform the Three Bedside A's (armband, allergies, assessments).
√   Document all medications after the patient has received them.

     Assignment: You have been assigned to administer medications to Tommy Douglas, Room 302. Floor: Pediatrics. Period of Care 2: 1115–1200.

   1. List all the medications the patient is receiving.

     2. Look up each medication in the Drug Guide provided.

     3. Which medications are antiinfectives? Is the dose appropriate for the patient's age and diagnosis?

     4. Why is he receiving this antiinfective?

Pacific View Regional Hospital	MRN: 1868054		Room: 401
	Patient: Harry George		
6475 E. Duke Avenue	Sex: Male		Age: 54
	Physician: Howard Steele, M.D.		

Physician's Orders

Weight: 143 lbs   **Age:** 54

Day/Time	Orders	Signature
Tue 0800	**Order Type:** General	*Howard Steele, M.D.*
	1. Change Cefotaxime to Ceftazidime 2 g IV every 8 hours.	
	2. Clean left foot wound with Normal saline, wipe dry with sterile gauze, then apply occlusive dressing to open area three times a day.	
	3. Please have physical therapist evaluate patient.	
	4. New lab orders today: Folic acid level. Repeat CBC and electrolytes. Amylase and lipase. Schedule bone scan of left foot for today.	

Pacific View Regional Hospital	MRN: 1868054	Room: 401
	Patient: Harry George	
6475 E. Duke Avenue	Sex: Male	Age: 54
	Physician: Howard Steele, M.D.	

Physician's Orders

Weight: 145 lbs   **Age:** 54

Day/Time	Orders	Signature
Mon 1830	**Order Type:** General	Howard Steele, M.D.
	1. Admit to Medical Unit.	
	2. Vital signs every 4 hours.	
	3. Send culture and sensitivity of wound if not done in ED.	
	4. Blood cultures from two different sites if T >102 F.	
	5. Foley catheter to gravity drainage.	
	6. Activity: Bedrest.	
	7. Keep left foot elevated on two pillows.	
	8. Have Wound Care Team evaluate left foot wound.	
	9. Do dressing changes per Wound Care Team orders.	
	10. IV of Normal saline at 125 mL/hr.	
	11. Continue Cefotaxime 1 g every 6 hours (started in ED).	
	12. Gentamicin 20 mg IV every 8 hours. Draw peak and trough with 5th dose.	
	13. Chlordiazepoxide hydrochloride 50 mg IV every 4-6 hours prn agitation.	
	14. Thiamine 100 mg PO or IM on admission and then daily.	
	15. 1800 calorie ADA diet.	

→ Proceed to Room 401, Harry George. Floor: Medical-Surgical. Period of Care 1: 0730–0815.

5. *Critical Thinking:* Review the patient's chart, including which medications the patient received in the emergency room. What *antibiotic* did he receive in the ER? Next proceed to the medication room and prepare his IV antibiotic for administration during this period of care. Compare the medications in the small volume IV storage bin with the MAR. Describe what potential medication error can occur related to the available antibiotics.

NAMING, SHAMING, AND BLAMING

Patients are admitted to the hospital with the understanding that they will receive quality health care, with the expectation of health improvement or relief from pain. Patients do not enter the hospital with the expectation of being harmed by the people providing their care.

Health care is a system. It operates by administrative layers and chains of command. With regard to medications, we have seen that it also functions by a *drug therapy chain*. We have seen that errors can occur at any point in this drug therapy chain, which can ultimately lead to medication errors and patient harm. When this happens, the institution investigates the error and strives to determine where the error occurred. What led to the mistake? Who is ultimately to blame for the patient being harmed?

The nurse, being the last link in the drug therapy chain, is the one most often placed "at blame."

Other industries label this narrow focus as the "sharp end." It ignores the bigger picture and uses the nurse as the scapegoat, focusing on a very small piece of the puzzle. Remember that the nurse is only *one link* in the drug therapy chain. It is estimated that there are between 20 and 40 steps and multiple hands involved in the delivery of a medication. Therefore, medication errors are more typically a "system failure" rather than an individual failure. A nurse is functioning in a "system" of health care and, without changes to the system, errors will continue to grow. Should the hospital have mandatory yearly medication review courses for all medication nurses? Should all high-alert medications be stored only in the pharmacy? Should a pharmacist be on duty 24 hours to avoid the need for the nursing supervisor to obtain drugs he or she may not be familiar with? These are all examples of system changes that may aid in the reduction of medication errors.

When a nurse discovers an error he or she has made or sees an error someone else has made, the nurse may be reluctant to report the error, thinking: "No one was harmed this time. Let's keep it to ourselves." Because health care can be punitive to the person who administered the wrong medication, it is often "safer" to keep quiet. As long as this punitive nature exists, **_underreporting_** will continue.

Without accurate reporting, it is impossible to see what link in the chain actually caused the error and impossible to make system changes that will improve safety. The cycle goes on, and the errors continue.

Other industries plagued by safety concerns have had great success by developing a "system approach." In air travel, for example, if an incident occurs, the first question considers not "who" caused the problem but "what" caused the problem.

Nurses need to be encouraged to be "whistle blowers" when they detect safety problems and should be rewarded when they identify potential errors. Until the institutions embrace the bedside nurses and their recommendations, "medication misadventures" will continue to rise.